Recent Advances in

Otolaryngology 9

W0246329

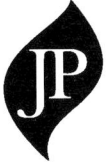

Recent Advances in

Otolaryngology 9

Holger Sudhoff MD PhD FRCS FRCPath
Professor and Chairman, Department of Otorhinolaryngology
Bielefeld Academic Teaching Hospital
Bielefeld, Germany

Mahmood Bhutta DPhil FRCS (ORL-HNS)
Clinical Lecturer and Specialist Registrar, UCL Ear Institute and
University College London Hospitals
London, UK

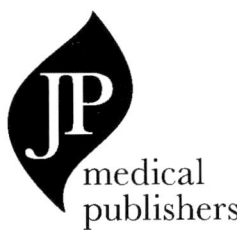

JP
medical
publishers

London • Philadelphia • Panama City • New Delhi

© 2015 JP Medical Ltd.
Published by JP Medical Ltd,
83 Victoria Street, London, SW1H 0HW, UK
Tel: +44 (0)20 3170 8910   Fax: +44 (0)20 3008 6180
Email: info@jpmedpub.com   Web: www.jpmedpub.com

ISBN: 978-1-907816-89-5

British Library Cataloguing in Publication Data
A catalogue record for this book is available from the British Library

Library of Congress Cataloging in Publication Data
A catalog record for this book is available from the Library of Congress

Commissioning Editor: Steffan Clements
Editorial Assistant: Sophie Woolven
Design: Designers Collective Ltd

Indexed, copy-edited, typeset, printed and bound in India.

Preface

The speciality of otolaryngology continues to develop rapidly. When we were compiling this volume of some of the recent advances in our field, the difficulty for us as editors was not which topics to include, but which to leave out. Advances in our specialty are testament to the initiative and dedication of our colleagues from around the globe, but we also recognise that some of these advances have been enabled by parallel advances in technology, engineering and biological techniques.

This collection of essays summarises the new: from a better understanding of the aetiology of disease, to the application of novel therapies. Chapters 2 and 5 describe new concepts in disease pathogenesis: the role of stem cells in the development of head and neck malignancy, and the role of hypoxia signalling in driving chronic inflammation in the middle ear. Chapter 7 discusses the relatively new entity of superior canal dehiscence syndrome: its diagnosis and current treatment. In Chapters 1 and 3, two new diagnostic and staging methods for head and neck cancer are described: optical diagnostics and PET-CT. We also have new and promising methods for treatment, some at the preclinical stage, some clinically established. These include vestibular implants (Chapter 9), audiovestibular regeneration (Chapter 8), Eustachian balloon tuboplasty (Chapter 6), middle ear implants (Chapter 4), and the medical treatment of lymphatic and vascular malformations (Chapter 10).

Recent Advances in Otolaryngology 9 is essential reading for trainees and practising ENT surgeons wanting to remain up-to-date with the latest developments in their field.

Mahmood Bhutta
Holger Sudhoff
December 2014

Contents

Chapter 1

Optical diagnostics in head and neck cancer

Taranjit S Tatla, Adrian Gh Podoleanu, Daniel S Elson

INTRODUCTION

Head and neck cancer is a heterogeneous group of cancers affecting a variety of distinct anatomical subsites in this region. Although they are composed of multiple tumour types presenting at varying stages of progression, the majority of head and neck cancers (>90%) are squamous cell carcinoma (SCC), arising from the epithelial membranes of particularly the larynx, oral cavity and oropharynx [1].

A multistep carcinogenesis model has been proposed to account for the aetiology and natural history of head and neck cancer development, mucosal cells progressing step-wise from mild, moderate, severe dysplasia, through carcinoma in situ, before invasion through the basement membrane into deeper submucosal tissue (invasive SCC). The diagnosis of early stage precancer/dysplastic pathological changes in biological tissues is fundamental to early clinical diagnosis and efficacious, lower cost treatment. The gold standard to date has remained invasive, tissue biopsy (under local or general anaesthesia) for histopathological characterisation. This is a time and resource hungry process, involving significant cost to the patient (waiting times, pain and potential functional deficit, as well as anxiety awaiting the biopsy result) and to the health care system (super-added material and manpower costs from additional steps in the patient pathway) including hospital admission for biopsy, tissue histopathological processing with paraffin embedding, sectioning, staining and trained specialist reporting with its inherent inaccuracy resulting from intra- and interobserver variation [2].

In recent years, 'optical biopsy' has been coined as a phrase through the development of various light-based imaging technologies, explored primarily to date as research tools in laboratories or in preclinical environments [3]. A wealth of ex vivo and in vivo animal and human data has emerged over the last decade on a number of optical technologies and tools related to disease diagnostics (cancer and noncancer). Optical biopsies can be acquired through different modalities, each with its own mechanism of action and requiring different modes of data analysis. They aim to provide a real-time, noninvasive and

Taranjit S Tatla BSc (Hons), MBBS, DLO, FRCS (ORL-HNS), Consultant ENT – Head and Neck Surgeon, North West London Hospitals, NHS Trust, London, UK. Email: ttatla@nhs.net (for correspondence)

Adrian Gh Podoleanu DiplEng, PhD, PGCHE, Professor, Biomedical Optics, University of Kent, Canterbury, UK

Daniel S Elson MSci (Hons), PhD, Reader in Surgical Imaging, Imperial College, London, UK

in situ optical signature of tissue with the possibility to transform diagnostic and clinical pathways for the head and neck cancer patient. They provide the prospective to render the need for intraoperative frozen sections obsolete. They also present the potential to guide accurate and precision-based resection with improved margins of cancer clearance, which should translate into better survival and reduced functional morbidity from treatment.

As confidence has emerged in the accuracy and utility of such techniques, more and more in vivo studies are being reported on the potential clinical effectiveness of these technologies for disease management in humans. Optical technologies are emerging that may not only detect head and neck cancer, but also direct stratified personalised medicine strategies through minimally invasive treatment modalities (transoral laser surgery, transoral robotic surgery, photodynamic therapy) and in the future aid the activation of emergent targeted therapeutic devices developed by the rapidly expanding field of nanotechnology.

THE EVOLUTION OF OPTICAL DIAGNOSTICS

The use of optical methods to aid diagnosis of different disease states is ancient when considering the colour and textural appearance of tissue, although within the last few decades a large range of new optical and biophotonics techniques have been developed that exploit light–tissue interactions to contrast disease states. This has been facilitated by the availability and reduced cost of optical components (e.g. lasers, light emitting diodes, optical fibres and charge-coupled devices), as well as the ability to miniaturise instruments to produce more portable devices that can enter the clinical arena of the physician's office or surgeon's operating theatre. The huge potential for such optical imaging tools, if demonstrated clinically for diagnostic accuracy (sensitivity and specificity) approaching the present histopathology gold standard, has encouraged the emergence of multidisciplinary groups for development and clinical translation of these technologies [4]. The field of biophotonics at present offers numerous choices of instruments for potential future routine clinical use, including on the one hand devices that are clinically proven to varying degrees of validity and already commercialised, and on the other hand, promising research tools that are in need of validation and development.

Optical imaging technologies in head and neck cancer have typically evolved to provide adjunctive endoscopic information to that provided by white light alone, to aid the clinician in both diagnostic and microtherapeutic management of diseased tissue. Illustration of clinical utility for disease diagnosis, cancer screening and surveillance, as well as aiding stratification and personalised therapeutic strategies, remain medium and long-term objectives [4].

Table 1.1 lists and **Figure 1.1** illustrates the spectral range of emerging optical imaging modalities that have been investigated in the context of head and neck cancer and a recent review [3] compares and contrasts the benefits of digital 'optical biopsies' taken by these techniques against conventional transmitted light microscopy. New technologies investigated in head and neck disease include narrow band imaging (NBI), optical coherence tomography (OCT), Raman spectroscopy, wide-field fluorescence microscopy and confocal microscopy, amongst others. Many of these are able not only to offer imaging at high resolution noninvasively but also allow users to interrogate molecular events and better image live cells without disruption of tissue. The role of the pathologist is evolving, going from interpreting tissue biopsy samples to acquiring, managing and possibly interpreting these high-resolution digital images, with the aid of appropriate software development and powerful computer processing.

Table 1.1 Comparison and contrast of optical modalities for head and neck cancer			
Method	Principle of operation	Field of view (FOV), resolution and penetration depth	Comments
Optical coherence tomography (OCT)	Reflections from different tissue layers are detected via coherence gate principles [8] to construct an A-scan, and scanning optics used to create B-scan images (cross sections) in real time	Minimum voxel size ~(3–20) x(3–20)x(7–20) μm Volumes up to 8 mm³ possible Maximum penetration depth: 1.5 mm	Limited penetration depth but enough to visualise epithelium (basement membrane violation in flat, nonexophytic lesions) and subsurface structures (cartilage etc) Three-dimensional architectural tissue detail but relatively lower molecular contrast compared to fluorescence imaging Can be combined synergistically with other optical techniques (i.e. confocal microscopy, fluorescence imaging, FLIM, Raman) in a hybrid assembly Adapting micro-optic components, to integrate OCT into catheters and needles, provides potential for deep-organ imaging inside the body (e.g. lymph node and thyroid nodule 'optical sampling') Fibre conduit affects polarisation properties
Confocal microscopy	Laser light is focused into the tissue and fluorescence is detected via a confocal pinhole to reject out-of-focus light. Beam is scanned to create an en face depth-resolved image	Minimum voxel size ~1 x 1 x 0.35 μm³ Volumes up to 1 mm³ possible with loss of resolution Maximum depth 0.35 mm	Very limited image penetration depth (few hundred microns) and so basement membrane may not be imaged (particularly where mucosa is thickened) Requires high magnification interface optics necessitating close tissue proximity to almost touch Small FOV results in random sampling of tissue but cellular level detail in optical resolution and contrast Can be combined with other techniques (i.e. fluorescence imaging and OCT) in a hybrid assembly
Fluorescence endoscopy	Colour image based on local tissue differences in fluorescence intensity. Often an exogenous marker is used to enhance the contrast	FOV ~ 1–100 mm Pixel dimension ~FOV/1000 Low depth resolution, most signals from < 100 μm depth	Relies upon tissue fluorescence for optical molecular contrast rather than transmitted or reflected light Fluorophore signal used to create image Fluorescence signals are often weak, although multiple fluorophores can potentially be visualised simultaneously Image affected by tissue morphology, endogenous absorbers, photobleaching, and illumination intensity artefacts (direct impact on sensitivity and specificity of tissue diagnostics). Hyperkeratotic and other diseased mucosa does not allow penetration and transmission of the illuminating light and so neoplastic changes in the basal mucosal cell layer remain hidden. Vascular lesions (granulation tissue and telangiectasia) produce a similar reduction in green fluorescence to neoplastic lesions (resultant from absorptive properties of the heme molecule) and inflammatory necrosis/scar tissue too can unpredictably alter tissue fluorescence signal Wide FOV (when used in combination, may be useful as guidance technique to direct OCT imaging in diseased tissue)

Continued...

Table 1.1 *Continued...*

Method	Principle of operation	Field of view (FOV), resolution and penetration depth	Comments
Fluorescence lifetime imaging (FLIM)	Image based on local tissue differences in the exponential decay rate of the fluorescence from a fluorescent sample once the excitation is abolished	FOV ~ 1–100 mm Pixel dimension ~ FOV/1000 Low depth resolution, most signals from < 100 µm depth	Lifetime of the fluorophore signal, rather than its intensity, used to create the image (advantage of minimising the effect of photon scattering in thick layers of samples) Minimally affected by tissue morphology, endogenous absorbers, photobleaching, and illumination intensity artefacts making FLIM a more robust fluorescence microscopy tool for clinical application FLIM mapping useful to determine relative molecular composition (i.e. collagen and elastin levels) and so increase specificity in diagnosis compared to fluorescence alone
Narrow band imaging	Narrow band 415 nm (blue) and 540 nm (green) light beams designed to penetrate mucosa and submucosa in combination to provide high surface contrast and display the morphology of superficial capillary networks and subepithelial vessels	FOV ~ 50 mm Pixel dimension ~ FOV/1000 Most signal from < 100 µm depth	Microvascular alterations and subtle neoangiogenic changes associated with precancerous and neoplastic diseases are more likely to be visible in vivo to the trained clinician's eye (compared to white light use alone), facilitating differentiation of nonmalignant from malignant lesions Early clinical studies show sensitivity of 88.9% and specificity of 93.2% in detecting malignant lesions; reported significantly superior (12% improvement) compared to white light illumination alone (however limited study numbers and single-centre trial data) Need for independent, larger, multicentre, randomised prospective clinical trials
Raman spectroscopy	Molecular vibrational energy levels are probed by a laser, which results in a unique optical frequency shift (Raman shift), acting as a spectral signature	Often nonimaging with sensing area of ~1 mm diameter No depth resolution, most signal from < 800 µm depth	May provide high level of compositional detail about tissue Low signal strength requires long acquisition time and cooled cameras Tissue randomly sampled due to small sensing area Imaging difficult and time consuming. Complex data analysis required to extract diagnostic information
Photo-acoustic imaging	Absorption of light causes acoustic ripples that may be detected using US transducer	Resolution scales with depth and ultrasound frequency. High resolution (<10 micron) and ~mm FOV at ~mm depths. Lower resolution (~1mm) and few cm FOV at few cm depths.	Requirement for contact of ultrasound transducer detector with the tissue surface for efficient detection of US signals Large range of imaging formats and scales provides many different diagnostic opportunities but the contrast principally comes from blood absorption Technology is currently being developed to make Doppler measurements of blood flows and to study microvasculature Endoscopic methods are increasing in popularity

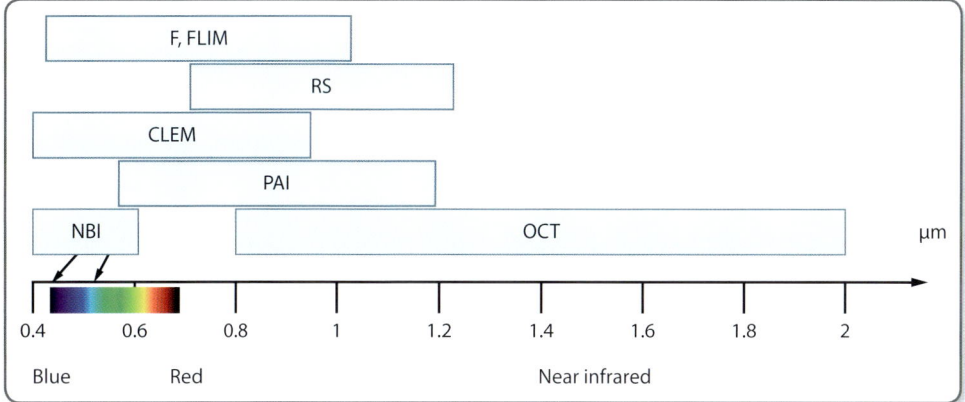

Figure 1.1 Spectral range of optical modalities used in head and neck cancers—the wavelength spectral range shown refers to the breadth of OCT in biomedical optics; the band around 1300 nm is the most commonly utilised and reported in Head and Neck tissue studies. CLEM, confocal laser endomicroscopy; F, fluorescence imaging; FLIM, fluorescence lifetime imaging; NBI, narrow band imaging; OCT, optical coherence tomography; RS, Raman spectroscopy; PAI, photo acoustic imaging.

NARROW BAND IMAGING

NBI is a commercially available, high-resolution endoscopic technique using contrast from blood vessels to aid diagnosis of dysplastic intestinal lesions which has recently been investigated in vivo for suspect oral and laryngeal lesions to differentiate precancerous and malignant laryngeal disease [5]. The technique is based on the fact that the depth of light penetration depends on the light wavelength; the longer the wavelength, the deeper the penetration. NBI filters the broadband white light of a xenon lamp into narrow band beams with two central wavelengths typically found in commercial devices of 415 nm (narrow band blue) and 540 nm (narrow band green) designed primarily to penetrate mucosa and submucosa. When used in combination, the two wavelength images provide high surface contrast, displaying the morphology of superficial capillary networks and subepithelial vessels respectively (**Figure 1.2**), from which clinicians are more likely to spot microvascular alterations in vivo to differentiate nonmalignant from malignant laryngeal lesions (**Figure 1.3**).

Ni et al. [6] reported their experience utilising consecutively white light and NBI system settings in vivo during office-based flexible nasendoscopy with topical local anaesthesia. They report sensitivity of 88.9% and specificity of 93.2% respectively in detecting malignant lesions through the addition of NBI, which they feel is significantly superior to white light illumination alone. They recommend its routine use for early detection of laryngeal cancer and precancerous dysplastic lesions.

Piazza et al. [7] emphasise that the larynx and hypopharynx represent an ideal site for NBI application because the thin, nonkeratinised, stratified squamous epithelium permits optimal visualisation of the subtle neoangiogenic changes associated with precancerous and neoplastic diseases. They advocate the routine use of NBI in different settings of laryngeal cancer management, from preoperative diagnosis and staging to intraoperative evaluation of microsurgical margins and post-treatment follow-up. They also advocate its use as an ancillary diagnostic tool for endoscopic management of patients with hypopharyngeal neoplastic disease.

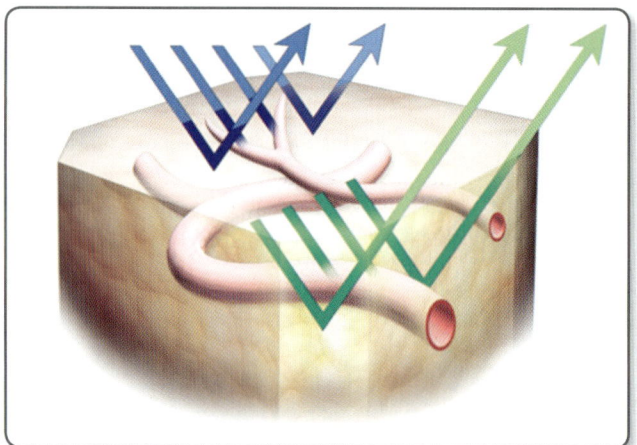

Figure 1.2 Absorption of narrow band imaging—narrow band light wavelengths of 415 nm (narrow band blue to interrogate mucosa) and 540 nm (narrow band green to interrogate submucosa) are used in combination to provide high surface contrast, displaying the morphology of superficial capillary networks and subepithelial vessels. Image supplied and reproduced with permission of Olympus.

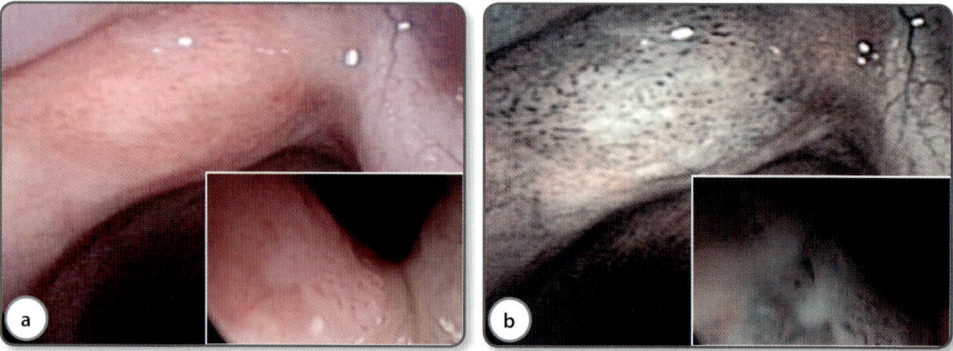

Figure 1.3 (a) Flexible preoperative videoendoscopy (up) and intraoperative view by 1200 rigid telescope (down) by white light high-definition television (HDTV) of erythroplakia involving the left vocal cord. (b) Same view by narrow band imaging (NBI)-HDTV (narrow bands 415 nm and 540 nm) shows better definition of lesion's margins and the typical vascular pattern. The histological examination confirmed the lesion to be carcinoma in situ. Images supplied by Dr Cesare Piazza at University of Brescia, Italy with permission of Olympus.

NBI study numbers presently are limited and larger, independent, multicentre and prospective clinical trials are required to validate diagnostic accuracy and clinical utility. Certainly relative to white light imaging alone, NBI adds clinically useful adjunctive superficial mucosal information. However, other optical techniques have been proposed which hold promise for even greater precancer/cancer diagnostic sensitivity and specificity. NBI may compliment these modalities, its advantages being relative low cost and ease in implementation.

OPTICAL COHERENCE TOMOGRAPHY

OCT [8] is an emerging technology first reported for cross-sectional retinal imaging in 1991. To date, its regular clinical use has been adopted mainly in the ophthalmology community, although with technological developments in the last 10 years, its potential for endoscopic application has been explored and potential adjunctive benefit slowly realised for multiple other organ systems including the larynx [4].

OCT uses low-power infrared light interferometry with collection of backscatter reflections at tissue layer interfaces. Up to micron level resolution of morphological detail is possible, allowing a penetration depth of 2–3 mm into tissue, equating to dimensions of standard excisional biopsy specimens for histopathology, but without the need for tissue removal. Its potential benefit as a diagnostic/therapeutic adjunct for office- and theatre-based clinical application in head and neck disease is slowly being realised as more and more preclinical and clinical studies are being reported [9,10–12]. Depending on the methodology (time domain, spectral domain or swept-source), OCT utilises a laser light source which may be broad bandwidth or narrow tunable. With time domain OCT (TD-OCT), interference signal is only observed when the path lengths of reference and sample arms are matched to within the coherence length of the light. By altering the position of the reference mirror to adjust the path length of the reference arm, the magnitude and time delay (corresponding to depth) of the reflected light from the sample can be measured. The contrast in OCT comes from the local variations in the index of refraction at the microinterfaces of various tissue layers as the optical beam scans the imaged tissue surface to provide two-dimensional (2D) (**Figure 1.4**) or 3D images.

The most successful OCT system to date, however, is the swept source OCT (SS-OCT) [8], which can achieve both highest acquisition speeds and sensitivity. The operation of SS-OCT is based on the demodulation of the optical spectrum at the output of the interferometer. **Figure 1.5** shows the main elements of a SS-OCT configuration. The spectrum exhibits peaks and troughs (channelled spectrum) and the period of such a modulation is proportional to the optical path difference in the interferometer. The optical source is tunable (swept source) and a photodetector is used to translate the channelled

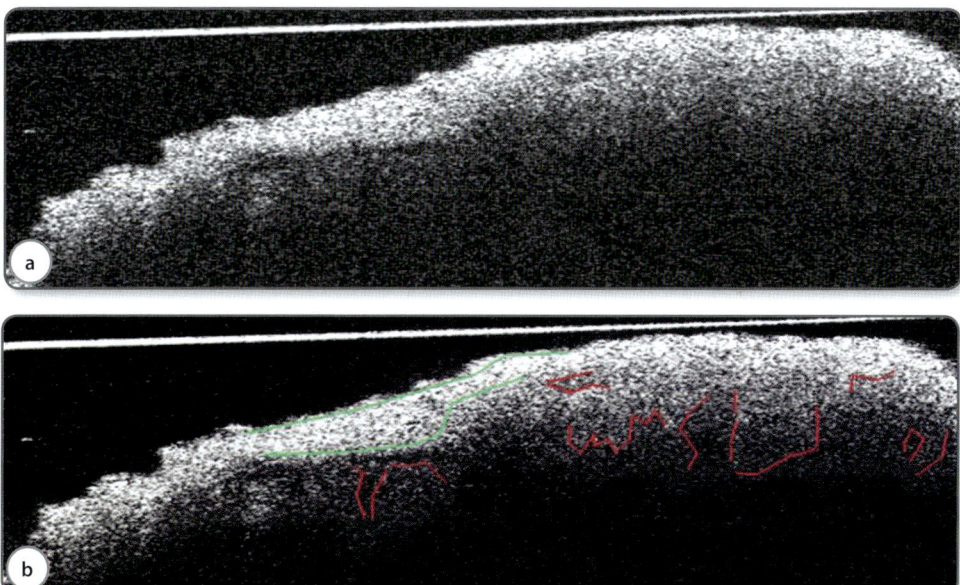

Figure 1.4 Axial B-scan ex vivo images of invasive laryngeal squamous cell carcinoma (SCC) taken with a 1300 nm time domain optical coherence tomography (OCT) imaging system by the authors at the University of Kent (Applied Optics Group). Red outlines (partial and complete) of dark OCT contours correlate with stromal epithelial transitions of well-differentiated SCC, whereas the green lines show bright OCT signal which appears to correlate with mature surface keratin.

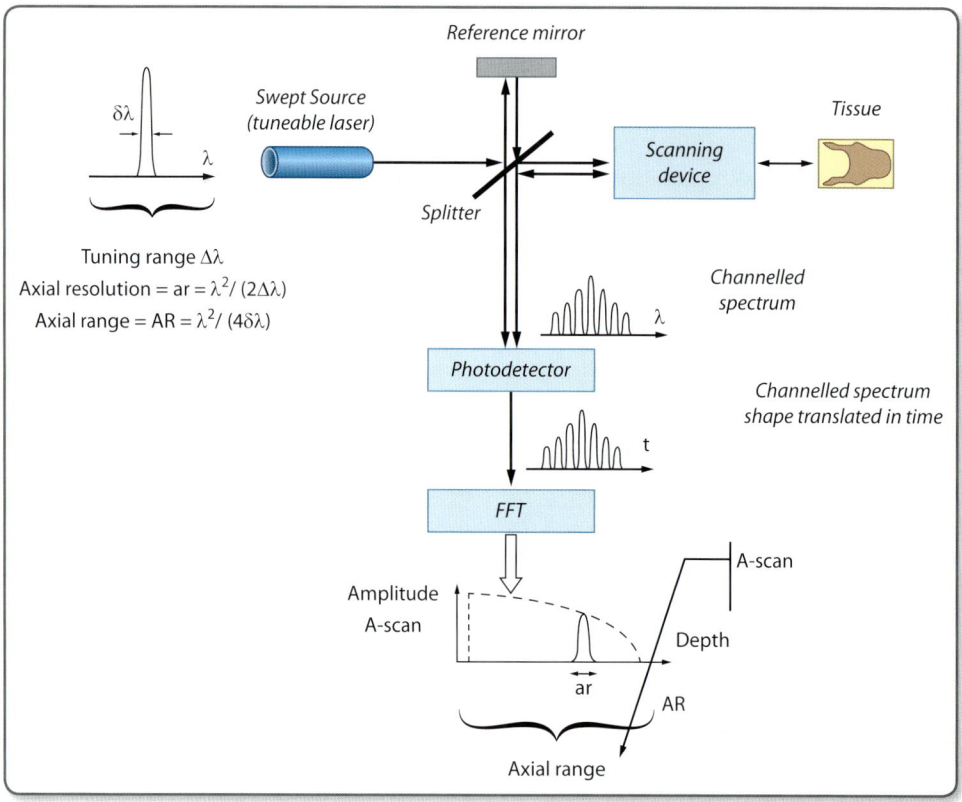

Figure 1.5 Optical coherence tomography (OCT) setup of a swept source OCT configuration. By collecting adjacent A-scans for successive pixels along a transversal coordinate using a scanning device, a cross-sectional image (B-scan, analogous to terminology used in ultrasound imaging) is obtained.

spectrum into a temporal signal. The larger the depth where signal is reflected from the tissue, the larger the number of peaks in the spectrum. Each scattering point imprints its own spectrum modulation periodicity, depending on its depth. A fast Fourier transform (FFT) of the photodetected signal translates the periodicity of the channelled spectrum into peaks of different frequency related to the depth position of the scattering centre, determining a profile of reflectivity versus depth (an A-scan). In the illustration, the channelled spectrum is shown for a single scattering centre within the depth range for simplicity. The spectrum width of the radiation emitted by the laser needs to be much narrower than the spectral distance between adjacent peaks in the channelled spectrum, and in practice, its finite width determines the axial range. The narrower the laser line, $\delta\lambda$, the larger the penetration depth. The larger the tuning bandwidth, the better the axial resolution, and values below 10 µm are easily accessible. Tuning speeds in excess of several MHz make the SS-OCT the fastest scanning OCT method.

OCT can reveal tissue microstructure and may be combined with confocal microscopy to achieve cellular resolution in the en face, similar to confocal endoscopy but with improved image depth (compared to confocal microscopy alone). Wong et al.[10] report in vivo experience using a handheld OCT probe in near or gentle contact with mucosa, for adjunctive examination of patients' larynges whilst under GA (comprising normal and benign laryngeal pathology), demonstrating and confirming the findings of ex vivo laryngeal studies [9] that OCT images compare favourably with conventional histopathology. The thickness of laryngeal mucosa in various subsites is demonstrated in detail with tissue architecture clearly displaying epithelial from subepithelial layers, integrity of basement membrane as well as microstructural features such as submucosal glands, ducts, blood vessels and cartilage. Benign true vocal cord pathology imaged included Reinke's oedema, polyps, nodules, papillomatosis, mucous cysts and granulation tissue. Others have added to this work, highlighting the ability of fibreoptic OCT to characterise basement membrane violation in invasive laryngeal carcinoma, as well as identifying tissue transition zones at premalignant margins of cancer. These findings were limited to superficial lesions as opposed to bulky exophytic growths where tissue penetration would be inadequate to allow the basement membrane to be seen. Just et al. [13] reported favourably on their unit's experience applying intraoperative OCT adjunctively to the operating microscope to define biopsy site location and resection planes precisely. Its potential for office-based application as an adjunct to flexible fibreoptic nasendoscopy for the awake patient under topical local anaesthesia has recently been demonstrated utilising a miniaturised endoscopic OCT probe passed in tandem to a flexible nasendoscope to view the larynx [11]. Rubinstein et al. [12] have recently presented their experience of intraoperative OCT imaging of benign and malignant disease conditions using the first commercially available OCT imaging system for upper aerodigestive tract imaging. This confirms the findings of earlier laryngeal OCT studies and provide further reliable intraoperative information to guide surgical biopsies, intraoperative decision making and therapeutic options for various pathologies including premalignant laryngeal diseases.

We have recently assembled a prototype dual SS-OCT instrument assembly to allow further investigation and validation of OCT clinical utility in an ENT-Head and Neck Surgery outpatient and theatre environment [4]. This portable and miniaturised assembly incorporates two distinct but inter-related instruments in the same assembly. Instrument 1 is dedicated to in vivo endoscopic OCT imaging of the upper aerodigestive tract based on an endoscopic probe head assembled by compounding a miniature 1D transversal flying spot scanning probe with a commercial fibre bundle 2D endoscope to facilitate simultaneous OCT cross-sectional mucosal images (B-scans) with en face fibre bundle white light endoscopic images. Instrument 2 is dedicated to either in vivo imaging of accessible skin and mucosal lesions of the scalp, face, neck and oral cavity, or ex vivo imaging of excised tissue biopsy specimens, based on a single OCT channel assembly incorporating better 2D interface optics in a handheld OCT probe. Following phantom model testing, in vivo clinical translation of this OCT technology is underway. Instrument 1 is under investigation as a possible endoscopic screening tool for early epithelial head and neck cancer. Larger size and better quality cross-sectional OCT images are produced by instrument 2, capable of acquiring a whole volume of the tissue. This provides a reference base for comparison and continuing research on imaging freshly excised ex vivo tissue, as well as in vivo interrogation of more superficial skin and mucosal lesions in the head and neck patient.

The potential, therefore, has been realised for a possible optical screening tool that has OCT as an integral and important component; either standalone to provide 3D micron-level morphological tissue detail and derangement with disease (e.g. loss/invasion of basement membrane in invasive carcinoma), or associated as a hybrid tool with other adjunctive optical imaging modalities that provide additionally some biochemical or functional discrimination between tissue and disease types [14].

Chen et al.[3] highlight additional advantageous clinical applications including the detection of premalignant lesions, identification of disease below the tissue surface, assessment of depth of tumour invasion, localisation of cancer margins, evaluation of effectiveness of therapy and reduction in the frequency and need for invasive biopsies, particularly during surveillance. In addition to these unique advantages that OCT provides for evaluating diseases present within the epithelial surface, advantages are gained by adapting micro-optic components to integrate OCT into catheters and needles to enable deep-organ imaging inside the body. In the head and neck, this may particularly find future clinical utility in lymph node and thyroid nodule 'optical sampling' in place of fine needle aspiration cytology [15].

Promising recent cadaveric work has illustrated the potential benefits of OCT use in assessment of tympanic membrane thickness as well as detection of spatial abnormalities at the micron range within the middle ear cavity [16]. We plan to progress this to in vivo application in the near future. Wang et al. have reported for cardiovascular applications the combination of highest achievable OCT acquisition speed with the smallest rotating engines that lead to over 3000 frames per second OCT imaging [17]. With further refinements of such probe tips, flexible OCT examination of larynx dysplasia and cancer becomes possible.

CONFOCAL LASER ENDOMICROSCOPY (CLEM)

Confocal microscopy increases optical resolution and contrast, with the potential to allow superficial mucosal tumours to be examined at high magnification in vivo, with en face cellular and histological detail revealed via the rejection of out-of-focus tissue layers. In recent times, commercially available confocal laser endomicroscopes have been investigated in vivo in the context of real-time, rapid and noninvasive image acquisition for mucosal cancer diagnosis by various groups [18]. By focusing a laser to a small spot size within the tissue and only detecting the reflected or fluorescent light from that spot by the use of a confocal image detector, light from planes above and below the plane of interest is rejected and better spatial resolution is achieved. By scanning the spot across the tissue and digitally reconstructing an image, an optical tissue section may be observed, analogous (albeit from a perpendicular plane) to a histological tissue section. The focal plane can be selected to see cells at different depths up to ~ several 100 µm before image quality becomes limited in practice. Most current applications require an exogenous dye such as fluorescein to be applied to the tissue prior to investigation and employ a grayscale display of the emitted fluorescence intensity.

In vivo CLEM trials in the head and neck are still awaited. Just et al. [19] report their use of confocal endoscopy intraoperatively to aid diagnosis and management of suspect cancer lesions using a custom-made scanner unit connected to a rigid endoscope. Although high-resolution images can be acquired rapidly and noninvasively, the systems are relatively high cost, provide small fields of view with image depth limited to a few hundred microns. This makes visualisation of the all important basement membrane, to make the distinction between high-grade dysplasia and early invasive carcinoma, highly unlikely and so limits the clinical utility of this technology for optical biopsy (as does the need for a tissue-touch technique). On the contrary, OCT provides a major potential clinical advantage over CLEM, that of nontouch imaging.

RAMAN SPECTROSCOPY

Various optical techniques are emerging with unique capabilities for molecular imaging based on the interaction of visible and near-infrared light with tissue. Each such technique interrogates a disease-specific source of contrast affecting one or more of the measurable properties of light [20]. This contrast may originate from endogenous or exogenous sources and be manifest in the wavelength, frequency, intensity or polarisation state of the measured optical signal. Raman spectroscopy is increasingly utilised as a research tool across a number of organ systems to spectrally characterise target tissue.

Raman spectroscopy (first described by Nobel prize winning Raman in 1928) [21] can provide information on the molecular composition and structure of a material by detecting and analysing the small amount of light that is inelastically scattered following interaction with molecules within the target tissue by monochromatic laser light (usually in the near infrared). The Raman spectra produced by this scattering reveal information about the vibrational state of the molecule, which is unique for each type of molecule. Raman spectroscopy has the potential to detect (noninvasively and in real-time) molecular optical signature change associated with tissue pathology.

Most studies to date have focussed on its potential with cancer diagnosis, whilst Stone et al. [22] reported promising preliminary data illustrating how Raman spectroscopy can distinguish normal laryngeal tissue and dysplasia from SCC, with sensitivity and specificity rates of 90% or more for detection of carcinoma. Lau et al. [23] have gone on to replicate some of these findings ex vivo, demonstrating good quality (high signal to noise ratio) spectral data collection in nasopharyngeal and laryngeal carcinoma specimens, as well as more rapid acquisition times. The same team more recently [24] has reported for the first time, in vivo human implementation of transnasal, image-guided Raman endoscopy to demonstrate good-quality Raman spectral data of nasopharyngeal and laryngeal tissue utilising a rapid 795 nm excitation Raman endoscopy system, coupled with a miniaturised 1.8 mm diameter fibreoptic Raman probe inserted down the spare instrument channel lumen of a medical endoscope. They report systematic Raman spectral dataset acquisition and cataloguing is presently underway for various disease states with a view to developing robust in vivo diagnostic algorithms for disease characterisation.

FLUORESCENCE ENDOSCOPY

Although fluorescence spectroscopy as a technique has been in use in various fields for over 100 years, its medical applicability for head and neck cancer detection has only recently come to the fore and been investigated [25]. Tissue autofluorescence is the natural capacity for tissue to fluoresce when exposed to light of a certain wavelength. Natural cellular fluorophores, such as flavin mononucleotide (FMN), exist as metabolic coenzymes in normal cells for aerobic glycolysis, but not in the anaerobic glycolysis pathways utilised by neoplastic cells [26]. Typically, filtered blue or ultraviolet light excitation of oxidised FMN and other natural cellular fluorophores in normal cells as well as structural proteins such as collagen, emits green fluorescence light which can be imaged and amplified by sensitive camera systems for display in real-time. Normal tissue appears green, whereas precancerous (dysplastic) or cancerous tissue does not autofluoresce or is covered by a thickened epithelial layer and appears darker (reddish/purple), with a possible increased red fluorescence originating from porphyrins [26].

Indirect autofluorescence laryngoscopy [26] and flexible autofluorescence endoscopy [27] have shown increased sensitivity for diagnosis of premalignant and malignant laryngeal lesions when used as an endoscopic adjunct to 'white-light' illumination, improving sensitivity levels to around 90% (a statistically significant increase of 12%). Others, such as Zargi et al. [28] showed specificity to be as low as 71%, due to some benign lesions displaying a loss of green fluorescence (i.e. benign hyperkeratotic lesions). Various groups have reported their findings exploring the potential additional benefits to autofluorescence in applying aminolevulinic acid (ALA) topically to the laryngeal mucosa, to preferentially induce fluorescence within neoplastic cells from porphyrins. Conflicting results have been noted as to whether ALA-induced fluorescence spectroscopy adds any further diagnostic accuracy to autofluorescence alone in the larynx, particularly in the context of laryngeal dysplasia and carcinoma [29]. However, the literature shows promise for autofluorescence as a technique with technical efforts now focussed on improving sensitivity and specificity (thus reducing false-negative and false-positive cases), as demanded by an accurate diagnostic tool.

Fluorescence lifetime imaging (FLIM) produces an image based on local tissue differences in the exponential decay rate of the fluorescence [30]. It can be used as an imaging technique in confocal microscopy, two-photon excitation microscopy, and multiphoton tomography with the lifetime of the fluorophore signal, rather than its intensity, used to create the image in FLIM. This has the advantage of minimising the effect of photon scattering in thick layers of samples. The time-resolved images from FLIM are thus less affected by tissue morphology, endogenous absorbers, photobleaching, and illumination intensity artefacts making FLIM a more robust fluorescence microscopy tool for clinical application (**Figure 1.6**). FLIM can potentially provide both high sensitivity and high specificity in disease diagnostics [31].

Marcu [31] has recently reviewed the available literature for ex vivo and in vivo application of fluorescence lifetime techniques for characterisation and diagnosis of biological tissues, concluding there to be a dearth of in vivo studies exploring time-resolved fluorescence spectroscopy and within those few reported studies, the numbers of clinical recruits remains small (20 or fewer patients). Nevertheless, the potential of this optical imaging modality as an accurate means of achieving optical molecular contrast in diseased tissues is highlighted for possible in vivo application in diagnosis of oral carcinoma. Sun et al. [32] have reported on a compact and portable FLIM system that has been designed and validated in vivo in a hamster oral carcinogenesis model. They found a significant contrast in fluorescence lifetime between tumour and normal tissues at 450 nm and an over 80% intensity decrease at 390 nm emission in tumour versus normal areas of the hamster oral cavity. This system has recently been applied endoscopically to image head and neck SCC (in vivo in man), which was found to have weaker fluorescence intensities and shorter fluorescence lifetimes than the surrounding tissues (**Figure 1.6**) [33].

PHOTO-ACOUSTIC IMAGING (PAI)

Photoacoustic imaging is a hybrid, non-invasive imaging technique combining the technologies of optical and ultrasound imaging [34]. Low energy, nanosecond pulses of laser light (usually in the visible or near-infra red spectrum) generate a photoacoustic

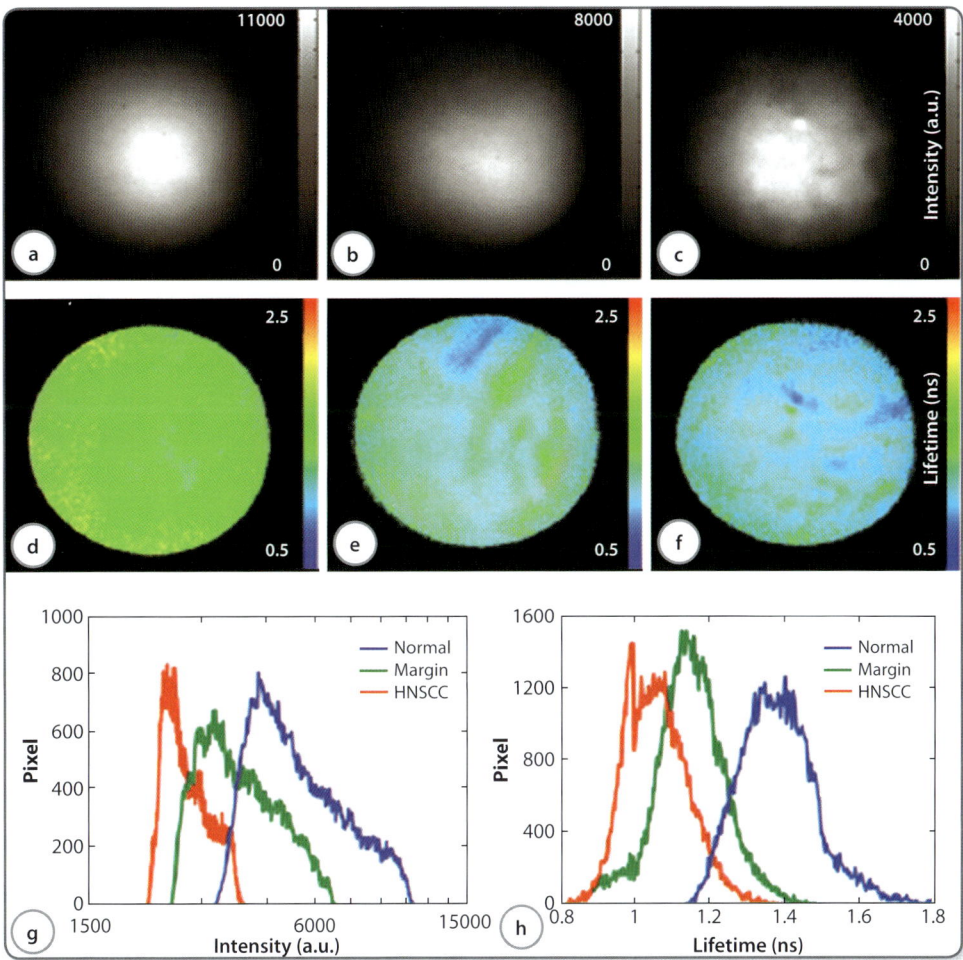

Figure 1.6 In vivo human autofluorescence and fluorescence lifetime imaging microscopy images of human buccal mucosa—parts (a–c) depict the intensity images, and parts (e–g) depict the average lifetime images from three areas: normal, tumour, and adjacent normal tumour, and their corresponding histograms are depicted in part (d) for intensity and part (h) for average lifetime. HNSCC, head and neck squamous cell carcinoma. Reproduced with permission from Cambridge University Press (Sun et al [32]).

signal from structures that lie centimetres deep below the body surface. Optical absorption in tissue is followed by localised heating and rapid thermoelastic expansion to generate ultrasound waves (photoacoustic waves). An ultrasound sensor on the body surface is used to detect these signals and an image of the location of absorbers within the tissue is calculated using a reconstruction algorithm. The images map the location and strengths of the tissue absorbers, with photoacoustic signal amplitude proportional to the optical absorption of the laser intensity by the absorber.

The technology provides a number of advantages over other optical imaging techniques, namely deeper tissue penetration (up to 5 cm), combined with potential for high contrast and resolution. For imaging superficial face/neck glands, such as thyroid/salivary gland nodules and cervical lymph nodes, there is significant potential being realised for head and neck clinical application. As a disadvantage in comparison with other optical modalities, collection of sound waves requires tissue contact, therefore in vivo applications demand further considerations for detection probes in terms of safety/disposal.

A number of head and neck specific studies have recently reported on ex vivo and in vivo experiments, utilising both endogenous molecular contrast, and exogenous, biomarker targeted contrast techniques.

Dogra et al.[34] have recently demonstrated in ex vivo human tissue, that multispectral photoacoustic imaging can allow differentiation between malignant and benign thyroid nodules, and normal thyroid parenchymal tissue. The technique appears sensitive to changes in tissue vascularisation (i.e. increased / abnormal angiogenesis, as is often seen in tumours relative to less vascularised normal tissue); the contrast is endogenous and is thought to be provided primarily by the key constituent deoxyhaemoglobin molecule. They have been able to demonstrate short acquisition times of 5 minutes for 3-D images measuring 45mm^3.

Levi et al. [35] too have focussed their attention on thyroid nodules, demonstrating the application of PAI in vivo in mice to help differentiate follicular thyroid cancer, through the use of an exogenous photoacoustic contrast probe targeting matrix metallo-proteinases (MMP-2 and MMP-9). These are two suggested follicular thyroid carcinoma biomarkers that have increased levels associated with minimally invasive follicular carcinomas, relative to follicular adenomas or multinodular goitre tissue (least expression). Both biomarkers are reported associated with follicular thyroid tumour progression and aggressiveness.

In vitro and in vivo oral cancer studies too have been reported in relation to the use of PAI, either using endogenous (label-free) or exogenous gold-nanoparticle labelled contrast. Laura Marcu and her team (Fatakdawala et al. [36]) have used the hamster oral buccal pouch carcinoma model to illustrate the complementary benefit provided by a multi-modal imaging system incorporating synchronous PAI (functional), FLIM (biochemical) and ultrasound back-scatter microscopy (structural) for enhancing in vivo detection of carcinoma, from pre-cancerous and normal mucosal tissue. The high PAI endogenous contrast signal is thought to be provided by high mucin concentrations around glands in the tissue (mucin is often over-expressed in carcinomas and exhibit high absorption at 532nm); they demonstrate for pre-cancerous tissue a complementary reduction in fluorescence lifetime. PAI was also shown to detect areas of high vascularisation within the tissue and tumour volume. Li et al.[37] have illustrated, through both in vitro and in vivo nude mice studies using oral cancer squamous cell lines, the potential for simultaneous, multiple selective biomarker targeting using antibody-conjugated gold nanorods. These act as exogenous contrast agents for photoacoustic molecular imaging with potential to aid cancer diagnosis. Yang et al.[38] have reported their favourable results of in vivo nude mouse PAI, illustrating chemotherapy-induced apoptosis in head and neck squamous cell carcinoma, using an exogenous near-infrared caspase-9 molecular probe. The results demonstrate the potential of PAI and this imaging probe to guide the evaluation of chemotherapy treatment in head and neck squamous cell. carcinoma.

DUAL/MULTIMODALITY HYBRID OPTICAL IMAGING FOR IMPROVING DIAGNOSTIC ACCURACY

In vivo optical imaging has the potential to interrogate tissue on a number of fronts simultaneously to provide complementary information using dual or multiple channels. No single optical imaging modality can measure all the possible clinically useful changes within diseased tissue. Multimodal optical characteristics together may act as a signature on the tissue's morphology, biochemistry, and biomechanics [14]. Multimodality systems combining OCT with multiphoton microscopy, OCT and fluorescence spectroscopy, OCT and multiphoton tomography, OCT and Raman spectroscopy and confocal Raman spectroscopy with confocal microscopy have been reported [14].

Park et al. [14] recently reported upon their development of a dual-modality OCT and FLIM system which simultaneously combines two complementary optical imaging modalities: OCT for 3D tissue morphology and FLIM for biochemical analysis. They developed a dual-modality system, comprising a subsystem (Fourier-domain spectral-OCT) linked to a high-speed spectrometer for subsecond, high-resolution volumetric 3D OCT data acquisition. This in turn is partnered to a multispectral FLIM subsystem based on a direct pulse-recording approach (upon 355 nm laser excitation), to provide 2D superficial 'fusion' maps of the tissue autofluorescence intensity and lifetime at three customisable emission bands with 100 μm lateral resolution. Both subsystems share the same excitation/illumination optical path and are simultaneously raster scanned on the sample to generate coregistered OCT volumes and FLIM images. In this report, they validated the system ex vivo using standardised fluorophore solutions and subsequently applied the system to characterise in vivo normal and cancerous hamster cheek pouch epithelial tissue. They correlated 3D OCT morphology of an epithelial cancer with corresponding standard H&E histology sections, characterising the normal epithelial tissue revealing the dominant fluorophore of collagen and cancerous tissue showing a different FLIM pattern due to the dominant fluorophore shifting to nicotinamide adenine dinucleotide (at 450 nm band) and shifting to flavin adenine dinucleotide (at 550 nm band) in the cancer tissue (**Figure 1.7**).

APPLICATION OF MOLECULAR BIOMARKERS IN OPTICAL DIAGNOSTICS

The clinical application of OCT and other endoscopic imaging modalities can be advanced further by utilising tissue contrast and spectral data provided by disease-specific biomarkers [39,40]. Molecular imaging capabilities are poised for clinical translation in coming years, providing adjunctive disease-specific information to improve further the accuracy of any 'optical biopsy' tool. Molecular imaging strategies fall into two categories: (1) endogenous molecular imaging, involving direct imaging of endogenous biomolecules; and (2) molecular contrast imaging, involving exogenous contrast agents introduced in vivo to bind specifically to biomolecules of interest. Contrast may involve near-infrared activated fluorescently labelled antibody probes, or indeed other labelling reagents coupled to antibody probes such as submicron microspheres or nanoparticles incorporating nontoxic materials such as gold or iron oxide [39]. At the present time, these remain

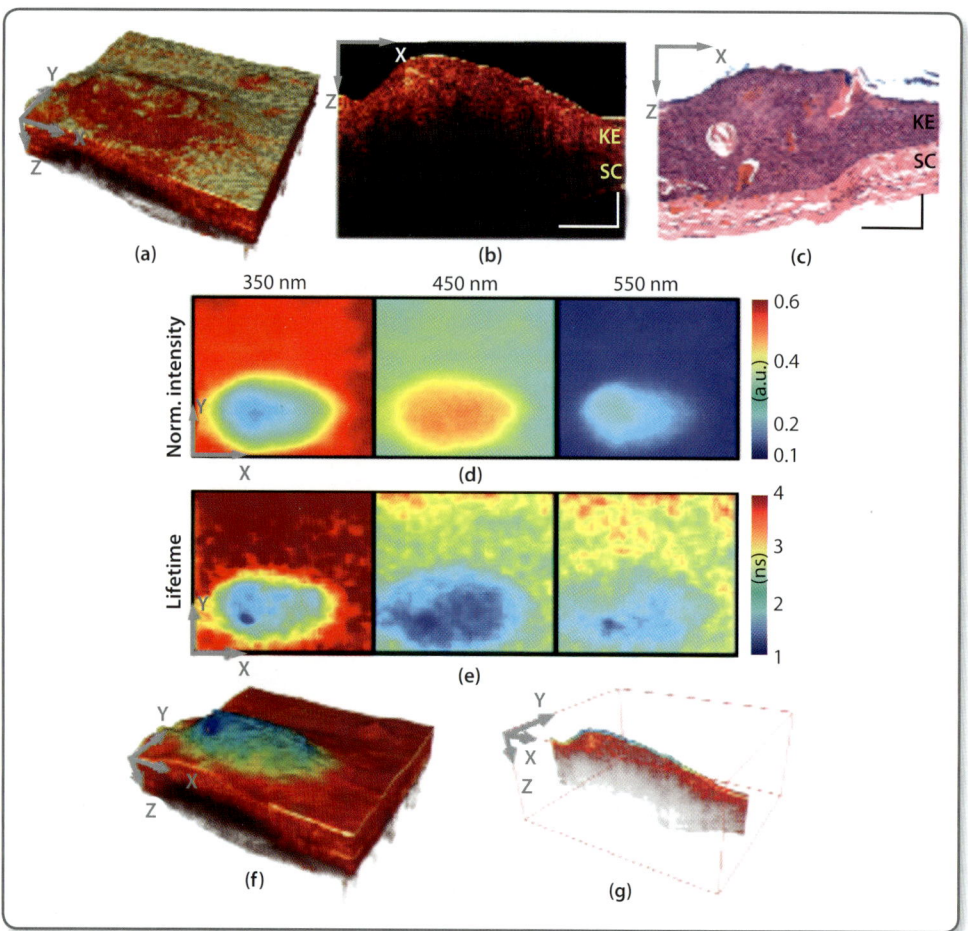

Figure 1.7 Dual-modal three-dimensional (3D) optical coherence tomography (OCT) images and fluorescence lifetime imaging (FLIM) maps of in vivo cancerous hamster cheek pouch [2000 (x) x 2000 (y) x 650 (z) μm]. (a) 3D OCT volume, (b) 2D OCT B-scan (KE, keratinised stratified squamous epithelium and SC, subepithelial connective tissue), (c) Haematoxylin and eosin histology corresponding to (b), (d) normalised fluorescence intensity maps, (e) fluorescence lifetime maps, (f) 3D OCT/FLIM volume with fluorescence lifetime in 390 nm band, and (g) orthosliced image from (f). Horizontal scale bar = 400 μm. Reproduced with permission from The Optical Society [14].

experimental and once validated ex vivo and in preclinical animal models, they will need to undergo human trials to assess their clinical validity and safety profile.

Multichannel endoscopes encompassing high-quality white light reflectance imaging associated with adjunctive near-infrared OCT and/or fluorescence imaging channels should soon become a reality for in vivo clinical use in the head and neck, as with other organ systems. In the context of oral/laryngeal dysplasia and head and neck cancer imaging, a number of potential biomarkers for optical diagnostics, 'optical beacons,' are presently emerging and are under investigation [41].

FUTURE DEVELOPMENTS

Advanced microscopy and optical imaging techniques are likely to evolve further with the progress of nanotechnology, facilitating ultra-high-resolution imaging and nanoscale sensitivity. The development of novel materials, devices and systems at the nanometer scale shall have far reaching potential for both nonmedical and biomedical applications; in the latter particularly for targeted drug delivery, molecular imaging, biomarkers and biosensors.

Various nanostructures (i.e. metallic, magnetic, liposomal and carbon based) are under investigation for innovative applications in medical and surgical practice [42]. Plasmonic gold nanoparticles appear to hold great promise amongst the various solid nanoparticles, nanotubes and nanocages for their possible diagnostic and tumour targeting application in head and neck cancer management. Gold nanoparticles have already been applied in therapeutic trials of cancers of the head and neck, in targeted therapy using tumour necrosis factor gold conjugate and in photothermal therapy [43].

Over the next few years, a continued and rapid evolution of optical diagnostics in head and neck cancer, as well as in other areas of ear, nose and throat disease is expected. Optical technologies will play an increasingly important role in the future design and control of nanodevices, to facilitate both ultra-fast and efficient optical tissue diagnostic arrays and molecular biomarker targeted application of nanotherapies.

Key points for clinical practice

- At the present time, the gold-standard and bench-mark for tissue diagnosis remains invasive biopsy and ex vivo histopathological examination
- Various optical imaging modalities have emerged over the last 10-15 years offering the potential for real-time, non-invasive, digital optical tissue 'biopsy' in vivo
- Translative research in optical tissue diagnosis of head and neck cancer, investigating the sensitivity and specificity of these various modalities either in isolation or in combination, is presently underway
- These techniques offer the potential for adjunctive benefit in diagnostic accuracy, to that afforded by modern white light, high definition camera imaging systems alone
- They also offer the potential for stratified, personalised medicine including precision 'smart' therapy (including trans-oral laser and robotic surgery), photodynamic therapy (PDT) and application of emergent targeted nanotechnology therapeutic devices
- All modalities exploit light-tissue interactions in order to contrast disease states and provide tissue detail
- Head and neck cancer studies are reported with narrow band (NBI), fluorescence/lifetime imaging (F/FLIM), optical coherence tomography (OCT), confocal laser endo-microscopy (CLEM), Raman spectroscopy (RS) and photo-acoustic imaging (PAI)
- Exhaustive and systematic correlative comparison is required with histopathology, in order to determine accuracy and clinical validity of these research tools
- Multidisciplinary international collaborative teams, including academics, clinicians, pathologists, physicists and engineers have emerged to progress this research and bridge geographical and professional divides
- There is likely to be rapid evolution of optical imaging application in head and neck cancer diagnosis and therapy, particularly with the emergence of nanotechnology

REFERENCES

1. Surveillance, Epidemiology, And End Results Program (SEER). SEER Stat Fact Sheets: All Cancer Sites. 2004-2010. http://seer.cancer.gov/statfacts/html/all.html Last accessed 13/07/13.
2. Fleskens SA, Bergshoeff VE, Voogd AC, et al. Interobserver variability of laryngeal mucosal premalignant lesions: a histopathological evaluation. Mod Pathol 2011; 24:892–898.
3. Chen Yu, Liang Chia-Pin, Liu Lang, et al. Review of advanced imaging techniques. J Pathol Inform 2012; 3:22.
4. Cernat R, Tatla TS, Pang J-Y, et al. Dual instrument for in vivo and ex vivo OCT imaging in an ENT department. Biomed Opt Express. 2012; 3:3346–3356.
5. Watanabe A, Taniguchi M, Tsujie H, et al. The value of narrow band imaging for early detection of laryngeal cancer. Eur Arch Otorhinolaryngol 2009; 266:1017–1023.
6. Ni X-G, He S, Xu Z-G, et al. Endoscopic diagnosis of laryngeal cancer and precancerous lesions by narrow band imaging. J Laryngol Otol. 2011; 125:288–296.
7. Piazza C, Del Bon F, Peretti G, Nicolai P. Narrow band imaging in endoscopic evaluation of the larynx. Curr Opin Otolaryngol Head Neck Surg 2012;20:472 doi:10.1097/MOO.0b013e32835908ac.
8. Podoleanu A Gh. Optical coherence tomography. J Microsc 2012; 247:209–219.
9. Bibas AG, Podoleanu AGH, Cucu RG, et al. 3-D optical coherence tomography of the laryngeal mucosa. Clin Otolaryngol. 2004; 29:713–720.
10. Wong BJF, Jackson RP, Guo S, et al. In vivo optical coherence tomography of the human larynx: normative and benign pathology in 82 patients. Laryngoscope. 2005; 115:1904–1911.
11. Sepehr A, Armstrong WB, Guo S, et al. Optical coherence tomography of the larynx in the awake patient. Otolaryngol Head Neck Surg 2008; 138:425–429.
12. Rubinstein M, Fine EL, Sepehr A, et al. Optical coherence tomography of the larynx using the Niris system. J Otolaryngol Head Neck Surg 2010; 39:150–156.
13. Just T, Lankenau E, Huttmann G, Pau HW. Intra-operative application of optical coherence tomography with an operating microscope. J Laryngol Otol 2009; 123:1027–1030.
14. Park J, Jo J, Shrestha S, et al. A dual-modality optical coherence tomography and fluorescence lifetime imaging microscopy system for simultaneous morphological and biochemical tissue characterisation. Biomed Opt Express 2010; 1:186–200.
15. Upile T, Jerjes W, Sterenborg HJ, et al. At the frontiers of surgery: review. Head Neck Oncol 2011; 3:7 (open access :http://headandneckoncology.org/contents/3/1/7)
16. Van der Jeught S, Dirckx JJJ, Aerts JRM, et al. Full-field thickness distribution of human tympanic membrane obtained with optical coherence tomography. J Assoc Res Otolaryngol 2013; 14:483–494.
17. Wang T, Wieser W, Springeling G, et al. Intravascular optical coherence tomography imaging at 3200 frames per second. Opt Lett 2013; 38:1715–1717.
18. Paull PE, Hyatt BJ, Wassef W, Fischer AH. Confocal laser endomicroscopy. Arch Pathol Lab Med 2011; 135:1343–1348.
19. Just T, Pau HW. Intra-operative application of confocal endomicroscopy using a rigid endoscope. J Laryngol Otol 2013; 127:599–604.
20. Pierce M, Javier D, Richards-Kortum R. Optical contrast agents and imaging systems for detection and diagnosis of cancer. Int J Cancer 2008; 123:1979–1990.
21. Raman CV, Krishnan KS. A new type of secondary radiation. Nature 1928; 121:501–502.
22. Stone N, Stavroulaki P, Kendall C, Birchall M, Barr H. Raman spectroscopy for early detection of laryngeal malignancy: Preliminary results. Laryngoscope 2000; 110:1756–1763.
23. Lau DP, Huang Z, Lui H, et al. Raman spectroscopy for optical diagnosis in the larynx: preliminary findings. Lasers Surg Med 2005; 37:192–200.
24. Bergholt MS, Lin K, Zheng W, et al. In vivo, real-time, transnasal, image-guided Raman endoscopy: defining spectral properties in the nasopharynx and larynx. J Biomed Opt 2012; 17:077002-1 to 077002-7.
25. Gillenwater A, Jacob R, Richards-Kortum R. Fluorescence spectroscopy: a technique with potential to improve the early detection of aerodigestive tract neoplasia. Head Neck 1998; 20:556–562.
26. Arens C, Dreyer T, Glanz H, Malzahn K. Indirect autofluorescence laryngoscopy in the diagnosis of laryngeal cancer and its precursor lesions. Eur Arch Otorhinolaryngol 2004; 261:71–76.
27. Mostafa BE, Shafik AG, Fawaz S. The role of flexible autofluorescence laryngoscopy in the diagnosis of malignant lesions of the larynx. Acta Oto-Laryngologica 2007; 127:175–179.

28. Zargi M, Fajdiga I, Smid L. Autofluorescence imaging in the diagnosis of laryngeal cancer. Eur Arch Otorhinolaryngol 2000; 257:17–23.
29. Hughes OR, Stone N, Kraft M, Arens C, Birchall M. Optical and molecular techniques to identify tumour margins within the larynx. Head Neck 2010; 32:1544–1553.
30. Chang C, Sud D, Mycek M. Fluorescence lifetime imaging microscopy. Methods Cell Biol 2007; 81:495–524.
31. Marcu L. Fluorescence lifetime techniques in medical applications. Ann Biomed Eng 2012; 40:304–331.
32. Sun Y, Phipps J, Elson D, et al. Fluorescence lifetime imaging microscopy: in vivo application to diagnosis of oral carcinoma. Opt Lett 2009; 34:2081–2083.
33. Sun Y, Phipps J, Meier J, et al. Endoscopic fluorescence lifetime imaging for in vivo intraoperative diagnosis of oral carcinoma. Microsc Microanal 2013; 19:791–798.
34. Dogra VK, Chinni BK, Valluru KS, et al. Preliminary results of ex vivo multispectral photoacoustic imaging in the management of thyroid cancer. AJR 2014; 202:W552–W558 (online).
35. Levi J, Kothapalli S, Bohndiek S, et al. Molecular photoacoustic imaging of follicular thyroid carcinoma. Clin Cancer Res 2013; 19(6):1494–502.
36. Fatakdawala H, Poti S, Zhou F, et al. Multimodal In Vivo imaging of oral cancer using fluorescence lifetime, photoacoustic and ultrasound techniques. Biomed Opt Express 2013; 4(9):1724-41.
37. Li P-C, Wang C-R, Shieh D-B, et al. In vivo photoacoustic molecular imaging with simultaneous multiple selective targeting using antibody-conjugated gold nanorods. Opt Express 2008, 16(23):18605.
38. Yang Q, Cui H, Cai S, Yang X, Laird Forrest M. In vivo photoacoustic imaging of chemotherapy-induced apoptosis in squamous cell carcinoma using a near-infrared caspase-9 probe. J Biomed Opt 2011;16(11):1160261-4.
39. Zysk AM, Nguyen FT, Oldenburg AL, Marks DL, Boppart SA. Optical coherence tomography: a review of clinical development from bench to bedside. J Biomed Opt 2007; 12:0514031–05140321.
40. Weissleder R, Mahmood U. Molecular imaging. Radiology 2001; 219:316–333.
41. Sadri, M, McMahon J, Parker A. Laryngeal dysplasia: aetiology and molecular biology. J Laryngol Otol 2006; 120:170–177.
42. El-Sayed IH. Nanotechnology in head and neck cancer: the race is on. Curr Oncol Rep 2010; 12:121–128.
43. Huang X, Jain PK, El-Sayed IH, El-Sayed MA. Gold nanoparticles: interesting optical properties and recent applications in cancer diagnostics and therapy. Nanomedicine (Lond) 2007; 2:681–693.

Chapter 2

Stem cells in head and neck cancer

Mark Prince

INTRODUCTION

An understanding of cancer stem cells and their relevance to the development and progression of head and neck squamous cell carcinoma (HNSCC) is essential to the creation of novel and more effective therapies for patients. The cancer stem cell theory of cancer has significantly changed our understanding of fundamental cancer biology and how cancers evade therapy and recur. In head and neck cancer, there has been little meaningful improvement in 5-year survival rates over the past 30 years, despite improvements in radiation, chemotherapy and surgical therapy [1]. The slow rate of change in these survival rates highlights the need for a substantial increase in our understanding of cancer biology and resistance to therapy

Stem cells have been of great interest to researchers, clinicians and patients for many years due to their potential to provide cures for many inherited diseases and for their ability to regenerate or replace diseased tissues and organs. However, due to their long life span normal stem cells or cells which acquire stem cell-like properties have recently been proposed to have the capacity to play a significant role in the development of malignancy. Unlike more differentiated cells which enjoy a shorter lifespan, stem cells are present from birth to death. The long time period over which stem cells survive provides the opportunity for the stem cells to acquire the number of genetic mutations required for them to acquire a cancer phenotype; whereas other cells are unlikely to be present long enough for this to occur. Additionally normal stem cells already possess a number of cancer-like characteristics including self-renewal, the ability to produce more differentiated daughter cells and an inherent capacity to migrate which may make their transition to cancer cells easier.

The concept of cancer stem cells has gradually evolved and gained acceptance over the past 20 years. Tumour initiating cells were first identified in haematopoietic malignancies. In 1994, Lapidot reported on the identification and isolation of cells that could initiate acute myeloid leukaemia (AML) when transplanted into an immunodeficient mouse model [2]. In 2003, a group led by M. Clarke isolated a highly tumorigenic subpopulation of cancer cells from breast cancer with the unique ability to recreate the original breast cancer in an animal model [3]. These cells were isolated from the other breast cancer cells using a panel

Mark Prince MD FRCS(C), Professor and Chief, Division of Head and Neck Surgery, Department of Otolaryngology-HNS, University of Michigan, Ann Arbor USA. Email: mepp@med.umich.edu (for correspondence)

of cell surface markers (CD24, CD44 and ESA). The other cancer cells were shown to have no or a very limited tumorigenic potential. These tumorigenic cancer cells were termed cancer stem cells. Subsequently cancer stem cells have been isolated from many solid tumour types including breast, brain, colon and pancreatic cancer. Cancer stem cells have also been isolated from head and neck cancer [4].

Cancer stem cells have the unique capacity to form tumours, recreate the tumour heterogeneity and self-renew. They also are proposed to be essential to tumour recurrence, contribute to resistance to therapy and to be responsible for the formation of regional and distant metastasis. Although there is still some controversy surrounding the cancer stem cell theory, the accumulating evidence from a large number of basic research and clinical studies supports the cancer stem cell theory of carcinogenesis [5,6].

Cancer stem cells represent a critical population of cancer cells responsible for cancer progression, metastasis and recurrence. The cancer stem cells must be eradicated or controlled in order for a patient to be cured of their cancer. Developing novel treatments directed against this important subpopulation of cancer cells has the potential to have a major impact on cancer survival rates.

CANCER CELL HIERARCHY

Normal tissues including skin, mucosa and the haematopoietic system are continually renewing and are hierarchically organised. At the top of the cell hierarchy in all tissues are stem cells from which the cells that maintain the tissues are derived. Normal stem cells have a lifelong capacity to self-renew (produce more stem cells) and to generate more differentiated daughter cells through symmetric and asymmetric cell divisions. Their more differentiated daughter cells have a limited or no potential for self-renewal. Normal stem cells are able to enter and exit a quiescent state and are resistant to cytotoxic agents.

Cancers seem to follow a pattern of hierarchical organisation similar to normal tissue [7]. This observation has led cancer researchers and cell biologists to hypothesise about the existence of cancer stem cells that would be at the top of the cancer cell hierarchy. Accumulating evidence supports the existence of cancer stem cells. Like normal stem cells, cancer stem cells are defined by a number of conserved biologic traits that are strikingly similar to those of normal stem cells. The cancer stem cell theory proposes that cancer stem cells can be isolated from the other cancer cells, represent a small subpopulation of the cancer cells, can reproduce the original tumour heterogeneity and are capable of unlimited self-renewal.

THE ORIGIN OF CANCER STEM CELLS

The cancer stem cell is defined by a set of traits, whereas the tumour cell that originates the cancer defines the cell type from which the cancer is derived. The initiating cancer cell(s) from which the cancer begins is determined by the first cell type to acquire a cancer phenotype through oncogenic mutations and epigenetic events [8].

Cancer stem cells could originate from any cell; however, normal stem cells are already capable of unlimited self-renewal, an essential characteristic of cancer stem calls. Normal stem cells also have a long life span that would allow them to acquire the genetic changes required for them to gain a cancer phenotype where more differentiated cells do not. These features make normal stem cells an attractive candidate for the origin of cancer stem cells. However, it is possible that cancer stem cells might derive from cells that are more differentiated if one of the first mutations or epigenetic changes that occurred resulted in a capacity for self-renewal. Recent work has demonstrated that self-renewal and pluripotency can be achieved through the activation of as few as four transcription factors [9]. This finding supports the idea that cancer stem cells may be derived from a variety of more differentiated cells not just normal stem cells or early progenitor cells

Currently the cell of origin for head and neck squamous cell cancer has not yet been defined. Although it is attractive to suggest that normal stem cells located in the basal layer of the mucosa provide the source for cancer stem cells for most head and neck cancers, this has not yet been proven. Work to identify the cell of origin for HNSCC will be important to develop treatments that can selectively destroy the cancer stem cells while preserving normal tissues and normal stem cells.

ISOLATION AND IDENTIFICATION OF CANCER STEM CELLS

The ability to separate highly tumorigenic cancer cells from the other cancer cells and for those cells to produce tumours in immune deficient mice, reproduce the original cancer heterogeneity and be passaged serially in an animal model (indicating a self-renewal capacity) is held to be the standard assay for the identification of cancer stem cells. Other potential assays to test for cancer stem cells include the ability of the cells to form spheroids when grown in low attachment serum free conditions are gaining acceptance as an alternate method to test for cancer stem cells but require further evaluation.

Cancer stem cells are typically isolated from other cancer cells in solid tumours by creating single cell suspensions of cancer cells and using fluorescence-activated cell sorting (FACS) flow cytometry to identify cells stained with fluorescence-conjugated antibodies of interest. A wide variety of cell surface markers and some biologic markers have been shown to be useful in isolating cancer stem cells from the remainder of the cancer cell population. Tumorigenic cells were first isolated from the other nontumorigenic cancer cells in AML [2]. This was followed by the discovery that cells with the surface markers CD34+/CD38– AML represented the tumorigenic subpopulation of AML cancer cells [10]. In 2003, M. Clarke et al. reported on the successful isolation of breast cancer stem cells with the cell surface markers ESA+/CD44+/CD24low/– from pleural effusions. As few as a hundred of these cells were able to establish tumours in an immunocompromised mouse model, whereas the other cells could not [3]. This was the first report of the isolation of cancer stem cells from a solid tumour. Since then cancer stem cells have been isolated from many solid and haematopoietic cancers using a variety of cell surface markers including HNSCC.

Interestingly some studies have reported the existence of overlapping or sometimes nonoverlapping populations of cancer stem cell populations isolated from the same cancer type including HNSCC using different cell surface or biologic markers [11,12]. This finding could be due to several possible factors. Different cancer stem cell clones might exist within the same cancer resulting in different cell surface marker expression. It is also possible that the tumour niche might be responsible for differences in cancer stem cell phenotype within area of the cancer and therefore different cancer stem cell marker expression within the same tumour. Finally, simple differences in experimental methodology may be responsible. If different cancer stem cell clones, potentially with differing attributes, can be found within the same cancer, this will greatly complicate the search for effective anticancer stem cell therapies. In HNSCC, the importance of the various cancer stem cell markers that have been reported to cancer stem cell behaviour is not yet known.

CD44

CD44 is a cell surface marker that has been reported to be useful in isolating cancer stem cells from HNSCC. CD44 is a large cell surface glycoprotein that is involved in cell adhesion and cell migration through its binding to hyaluronic acid and other extracellular ligands. Post-transcriptional and translational modifications allow CD 44 to bind to growth factors and metalloproteinase MMP9 that results in a wide range of functions including aiding the adherence of leukocytes to endothelial cells, inhibition of apoptosis and the invasion and subsequent metastasis of cancer cells [13].

Head and neck cancer cells that express high levels of CD44 have been characterised as having a more primitive cellular morphology, and increased expression of known stem cell markers, such as BMI-1 [4]. A number of studies have indicated that CD44 expression can isolate highly tumorigenic cells from HNSCC that are resistant to therapy, more invasive and have the ability to form distant metastasis [14,15]. CD 44 has a number of different isoforms. Work performed by Wang et al. in 2009 revealed that isoforms v3, v6 and v10 were associated with tumour stage, the presence of metastasis and reduced disease free survival [13]. The relevance of CD44 isoforms to cancer stem behaviour has not yet been elucidated.

Despite the reports indicating the usefulness of CD44 as a marker for cancer stem cells in head and neck cancer, it has some limitations. All head and neck cancer cells express CD44 to some degree, making the selection process dependent on the skill of the researcher to isolate the cancer cells with the highest CD44 expression levels. CD 44 is also expressed in many normal cells including head and neck epithelium. Further work needs to be performed to better characterise the usefulness of CD44 expression as a cancer stem cell marker in HNSCC and to better define the role CD44 expression may have in cancer stem cell behaviour.

Aldehyde dehydrogenase

Aldehyde dehydrogenase (ALDH) is a highly conserved intracellular enzyme. ALDH represents an important cellular defence capable of catalysing the oxidation of aldehydes in physiologic and pathologic cellular processes. ALDH1A1 and ALDH3A1 are two isoforms of ALDH that have an important role normal stem cell physiology. ALDH has been shown to be a marker for cancer stem cell in haematologic and solid organ malignancies including head and neck cancer [11,12] (**Figure 2.1**). The ability of high levels of ALDH activity to be used to isolate normal haematopoietic stem cells, embryonic stem cells and stem cells from many solid tumours suggests it may represent a highly maintained stem cell marker.

HNSCC cells with high levels of ALDH expression have been shown to be highly tumorigenic, capable of producing tumours with as few as 500 cells in a NOD/SCID animal model. ALDH1+ HNSCC cells have also been shown to create spheroids, have a greater invasive capacity and are resistant to radiation therapy. There is overlap between the ALDH expressing cancer cells and CD44+ cells, but their relationship is yet to be fully investigated in HNSCC [12].

Side population

The side population (SP) assay is another method of identifying stem cell populations. The SP of cells is isolated from other cells based on their ability to efflux the fluorescent DNA binding dye Hoechst 33342. This ability is related to ABCG2 transporter gene activity, which is known to be active in normal stem cells. SP cells have been reported to be a source of

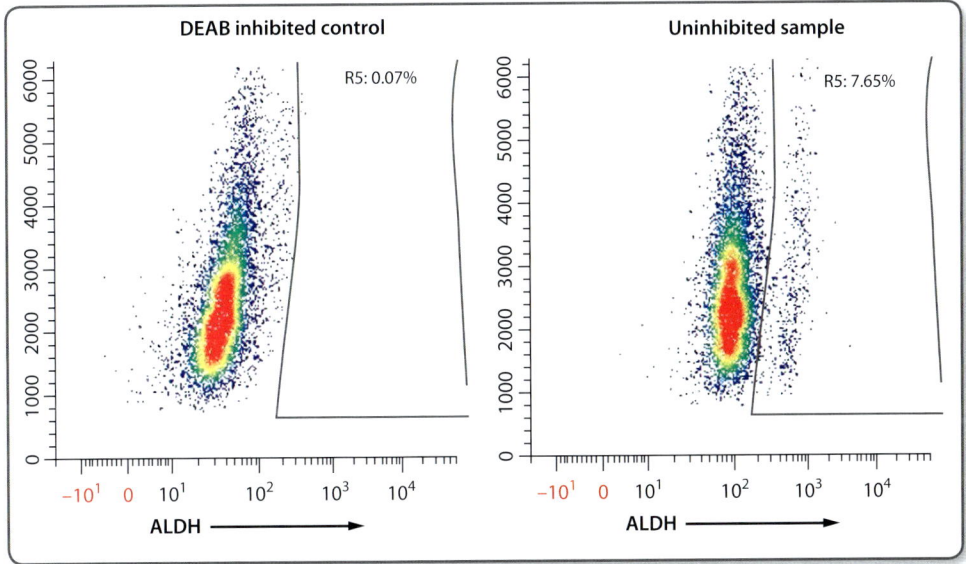

Figure 2.1 Head and neck cancer cells sorted for aldehyde dehydrogenase activity. (a) Initial fluorescence-activated cell sorting analysis is performed with diethylaminobenzaldehyde inhibition of aldehyde dehydrogenase activity. (b) Sorting is then performed and the cancer cells with high levels of aldehyde dehydrogenase activity can be isolated. In this case, the percentage of cancer stem cells in the sample is 7.65%.

cancer stem cells in a number of malignancies. Zhang et al. isolated SP cells from oral cavity tumours and found they had similar gene expression profiles to other cancer stem cell populations [16]. Similarly, SP cells isolated from a HNSCC cell line were reported to have a cancer stem cell phenotype [17]. The Hoechst 33342 dye is cytotoxic making this usefulness of this selection method potentially somewhat limited as it may affect cell survival or cell tumorigenicity assays.

CD 133

CD133 is a cell surface marker that has been reported to be a potential cancer stem cell marker for a variety of cancer types. Like CD44, CD133 is a transmembrane glycoprotein. CD133 is commonly expressed in haematopoietic stem cells, endothelial progenitor cells and other normal tissue stem cells. Several studies have reported that CD133+ HNSCC cells exhibit cancer stem cell characteristics including spheroid formation, tumour formation and increased clonogenicity. There have, however, been conflicting reports about the tumorigenic potential of CD133+ and CD133– cancer cell populations in other tumour sites that raise some concerns about its utility as a cancer stem cell marker [18,19].

cMet

cMet is a tyrosine kinase receptor for hepatocyte growth factor. It has been reported to be associated with metastasis and decreased cancer survival in head and neck cancer. cMet+ HNCSS cancer cells have been reported to be more tumorigenic than CD44+ cells. Cells that were positive for the combination of CD44+/cMet+ were more tumorigenic than ALDH+ cells [20]. Further investigation of single cancer stem cell markers and combinations of markers needs to be performed in HNSCC.

Cancer stem cell gene expression

The ability to separate cancer stem cells from the other cancer cells by flow cytometry has allowed for the study of gene expression in these cells. There has been particular interest in evaluating the expression of genes known to be associated with normal stem cells. A number of stem cell-related genes have been reported to be active in HNSCC, although their relevance to the cancer stem cell phenotype is poorly understood.

BMI-1 is a gene that is considered to be critical to the maintenance of stem cell self-renewal. Although it appears to be expressed in HNSCC, it has not been useful as a marker of HNSCC cancer stem cells [4,21]. Knockdown of BMI-1 expression in ALDH+ HNSCC cells resulted in significant reduction in self-renewal and radiation and chemotherapy resistance. BMI-1 expression promotes invasion and metastasis in ALDH+ HNSCC cells [21]. These results suggest that BMI-1 plays a key role in HNSCC maintenance and behaviour. As it is expressed in normal stem cells, it is unlikely to represent a useful therapeutic target.

Epithelial to mesenchymal transition (EMT) has been reported to be essential for HNSCC and other cancer cells to migrate and form metastasis [22]. Cancer cells must gain a mesenchymal phenotype in order to migrate effectively. Increased expression of Snail and Twist has been demonstrated in HNSCC cancer stem cells and has been correlated with outcome. The exact mechanisms regulating EMT in HNSCC cancer stem cells are unknown; however, evaluating known genes associated with stemness may rapidly advance our understanding of this critical process.

CLINICAL RELEVANCE

Treatment failure

Cancer stem cells are inherently resistant to current treatments including radiation and chemotherapy [20,23]. Surgery, although effective in removing all the cancer cells in the operative specimen, does not control cancer cells that are not removed and cannot control distant metastatic disease. Traditional measures of tumour response to radiation or chemotherapy are based on the percentage of tumour shrinkage and do not account for the proportion of cancer cells that remain, which have tumorigenic potential (i.e. the cancer stem cells). If even one cancer stem cell remains, under the right conditions, the cancer will recur. In order to account for the presence of cancer stem cells methods that can reliably and easily measure the effect of therapies on the cancer stem cell population need to be developed. This will be critical to our ability to measure the results of anticancer stem cell therapies that are developed.

In HNSCC, the proportion of CD44+ cells in a patient's primary tumour has been shown to be associated with patient outcomes. A study of patient with HNSCC revealed that the higher the per cent of CD44+ cells present in the primary tumour, the higher the likelihood of treatment failure [15]. It has also been reported that the presence of HNCSC cells expressing the cancer stem cell markers CD44, CD24, Oct4 and integrin-b1 was associated with poor outcomes following radiotherapy [23]. In laryngeal HNSCC, cells overexpressing CD133 and ABCG2 had a significantly reduced cell death rate when cultured with common chemotherapy agents [24]. Taken together these reports suggest cancer stem cells are more resistant to common therapies for HNSCC and likely are responsible for the treatment failures. It also suggests that efforts to change the cancer stem cell phenotype (by SNAIL inhibition for example) can change their sensitivity to current therapy.

Metastasis

Regional and distant metastases in HNSCC correlate with a poor prognosis with limited treatment options. Improved understanding of the processes that regulate the development of metastases may allow for more effective treatment of HNSCC patients with metastatic disease. Cancer stem cells have already been linked with the development of distant metastasis in breast cancer and in pancreatic carcinoma. In patients suffering from breast cancer, analysis of bone marrow has shown enrichment of cells expressing the breast cancer stem cell markers [25]. In pancreatic adenocarcinoma, a subgroup of pancreatic cancer stem cell expressing CD133+/CXCR4+ was shown to be at the invasive front and has an enhanced metastatic phenotype [26]. In HNSCC, there is increasing evidence that cancer stem cells may play a pivotal role in the development of metastasis.

As metastasis results from the spread of primary tumour cells through the blood stream or lymphatics, metastasis must be derived from circulating tumour cells. Circulating cancer cells are present in the blood of patients with HNSCC and have been shown to have prognostic importance [27]. The exact role of cancer stem cells in circulating tumour cells is unknown and will require further study; however, there is accumulating evidence that HNSCC cancer stem cells are critical to the development of metastasis (**Figure 2.2**).

Cancer stem cell-specific therapies

The idea of developing therapies that are able to specifically target and kill cancer stem cells is very attractive as evidence suggests that the cancer stem cell subpopulation of cancer cells is responsible for the treatment failures. Although current therapies are obviously

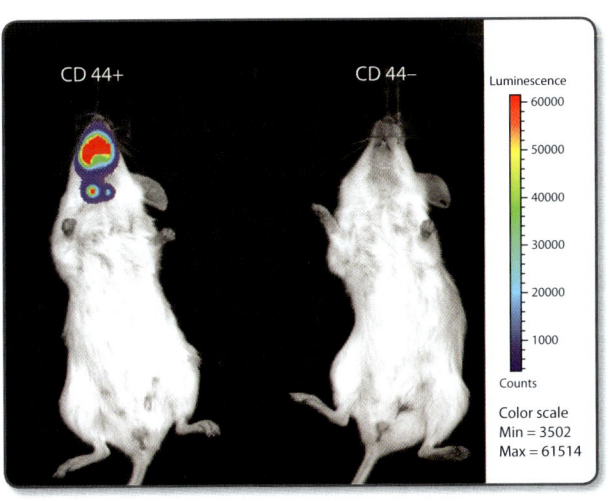

Figure 2.2 Head and neck cancer cells sorted for CD44 expression and implanted into mice demonstrating primary tumour development and the metastatic potential of the CD44+ cells.

effective in eradicating the cancer stem cells in some patients, in approximately 50% of patients with HNSCC who eventually succumb to their disease, it appears our current therapies are not effective in removing all the cancer stem cells. Methods that increase the cancer stem cells sensitivity to current therapeutic agents or new treatments that can specifically target the cancer stem cells are urgently needed.

Attempts have been made to target cancer stem cells through their biomarkers. Targeting CD44, which is also expressed by many normal stem cells, might produce unacceptable side effects. Utilising cancer-specific isoforms of CD44 might reduce the possible side effects; however, a phase one trial utilising an anti-CD44v6 antibody in HNSCC resulted in severe skin toxicity [28,28a]. Efforts to target the ABC transporter genes, which are active in cancer stem cells, were terminated because of concerns about the effect on the blood–brain barrier and normal adult stem cells [26]. Other treatments that might target cancer stem cell molecular pathways run the risk of detrimental effects on normal stem cell populations potentially limiting this therapeutic approach.

Recently, Li et al. [29] reported on the development of a dendritic cell-based anticancer vaccine that is directed against the cancer stem cell population. The results indicate that the immune system can be primed to recognise cancer stem cells and produce a meaningful humoral and cellular response [29]. This treatment represents a novel method to utilise the patient's own immune system to target the cancer stem cells and could have wide applicability to many tumour sites.

The development of treatments that can be directed against the cancer stem cell population is very complicated. As there is a large overlap in the molecular pathways that are important to both normal stem cell and cancer stem cell maintenance, therapy directed against cancer stem cells has the potential to have major deleterious effects on the normal stem cell population. Despite this evidence continues to accumulate that treatments that fail to efficiently destroy the cancer stem cell population will be ineffective in providing a cure for patients. Novel treatments or combinations of treatments against cancer stem cells must be developed to improve the rates of long-term cures for patients.

Key points for clinical practice

- Cancer stem cells are the highly tumorigenic population of cancer cells responsible for cancer growth and metastasis.
- Cancer stem cells can be isolated from solid cancers including head and neck cancer.
- Cancer stem cells have important biologic and behavioural differences from the other cancer cells.
- Cancer stem cells are an important target for novel treatments, as eradication of all cancer stem cells is critical to achieving a cure.
- Cancer stem cells and normal stem cells share many molecular pathways making the development of pathway specific treatments complex.

REFERENCES

1. Warnakulasuriya S. Global epidemiology of oral and oropharyngeal cancer. Oral Oncol 2009; 45:309–316.
2. Lapidot T, Sirard C, Vormoor J, et al. A cell initiating human acute myeloid leukaemia after transplantation into SCID mice. Nature 1994; 367:645–648.

3. Al-Hajj M, Wicha MS, Benito-Hernandez A, Morrison SJ, Clarke MF. Prospective identification of tumorigenic breast cancer cells. Proc Natl Acad Sci U S A 2003; 100:3983–3988.
4. Prince ME, Sivanandan R, Kaczorowski A, et al. Identification of a subpopulation of cells with cancer stem cell properties in head and neck squamous cell carcinoma. Proc Natl Acad Sci U S A 2007; 104:973–978.
5. Quintana E, Shackleton M, Foster HR, et al. Phenotypic heterogeneity among tumorigenic melanoma cells from patients that is reversible and not hierarchically organized. Cancer Cell. 2010; 18:510–523.
6. Huang SD, Yuan Y, Tang H, et al. Tumor cells positive and negative for the common cancer stem cell markers are capable of initiating tumor growth and generating both progenies. PLoS One 2013; 8:e54579.
7. Reya T, Morrison SJ, Clarke MF, Weissman IL. Stem cells, cancer, and cancer stem cells. Nature 2001; 414:105–111.
8. Visvader JE. Cells of origin in cancer. Nature 2011; 469:314–322.
9. Yu J, Vodyanik MA, Smuga-Otto K, et al. Induced pluripotent stem cell lines derived from human somatic cells. Science 2007; 318:1917–1920.
10. Bonnet D, Dick JE. Human acute myeloid leukemia is organized as a hierarchy that originates from a primitive hematopoietic cell. Nat Med 1997; 3:730–737.
11. Ginestier C, Hur MH, Charafe-Jauffret E, et al. ALDH1 is a marker of normal and malignant human mammary stem cells and a predictor of poor clinical outcome. Cell Stem Cell 2007; 1:555–567.
12. Clay MR, Tabor M, Owen JH, et al. Single-marker identification of head and neck squamous cell carcinoma cancer stem cells with aldehyde dehydrogenase. Head Neck 2010; 32:1195–1201.
13. Wang SJ, Wong G, de Heer AM, Xia W, Bourguignon LY. CD44 variant isoforms in head and neck squamous cell carcinoma progression. Laryngoscope 2009; 119:1518–1530.
14. Davis SJ, Divi V, Owen JH, et al. Metastatic potential of cancer stem cells in head and neck squamous cell carcinoma. Arch Otolaryngol Head Neck Surg 2010; 136:1260–1266.
15. Joshua B, Kaplan MJ, Doweck I, et al. Frequency of cells expressing CD44, a head and neck cancer stem cell marker: correlation with tumor aggressiveness. Head Neck 2012;34(1):42–49.
16. Zhang P, Zhang Y, Mao L, Zhang Z, Chen W. Side population in oral squamous cell carcinoma possesses tumor stem cell phenotypes. Cancer Lett 2009; 277:227–234.
17. Tabor MH, Clay MR, Owen JH, et al. Head and neck cancer stem cells: the side population. Laryngoscope 2011; 121:527–533.
18. Wu Y, Wu PY. CD133 as a marker for cancer stem cells: progresses and concerns. Stem Cells Dev 2009; 18:1127–1134.
19. Shmelkov SV, Butler JM, Hooper AT, et al. CD133 expression is not restricted to stem cells, and both CD133+ and CD133- metastatic colon cancer cells initiate tumors. J Clin Invest 2008; 118:2111–2120.
20. Sun S, Wang Z. Head neck squamous cell carcinoma c-Met+ cells display cancer stem cell properties and are responsible for cisplatin-resistance and metastasis. Int J Cancer 2011; 129:2337–2348.
21. Yu CC, Lo WL, Chen YW, et al. Bmi-1 regulates snail expression and promotes metastasis ability in head and neck squamous cancer-derived ALDH1 positive cells. J Oncol 2011; 2011.
22. Chen C, Wei Y, Hummel M, et al. Evidence for epithelial-mesenchymal transition in cancer stem cells of head and neck squamous cell carcinoma. PLoS One 2011; 6:2011.
23. Koukourakis MI, Giatromanolaki A, Tsakmaki V, Danielidis V, Sivridis E. Cancer stem cell phenotype relates to radio-chemotherapy outcome in locally advanced squamous cell head-neck cancer. Br J Cancer 2012; 106:846–853.
24. Yang JP, Liu Y, Zhong W, et al. Chemoresistance of CD133+ cancer stem cells in laryngeal carcinoma. Chin Med J (Engl) 2011; 124:1055–1060.
25. Balic M, Lin H, Young L, et al. Most early disseminated cancer cells detected in bone marrow of breast cancer patients have a putative breast cancer stem cell phenotype. Clin Cancer Res 2006; 12:5615–5621.
26. Hermann PC, Huber SL, Herrler T, et al. Distinct populations of cancer stem cells determine tumor growth and metastatic activity in human pancreatic cancer. Cell Stem Cell. 2007; 1:313–323.
27. Möckelmann N, Laban S, Pantel K, Knecht R. Circulating tumor cells in head and neck cancer: clinical impact in diagnosis and follow-up. Eur Arch Otorhinolaryngol. Eur Arch Otorhinolaryngol 2014; 271(1):15-21.
28. Riechelmann H, Sauter A, Golze W, et al. Phase I trial with the CD44v6-targeting immunoconjugate bivatuzumab mertansine in head and neck squamous cell carcinoma. Oral Oncol 2008; 44:823–829. 28a. Hermann DM, Kilic E, Spudich A, et al. Role of drug efflux carriers in the healthy and diseased brain. Ann Neurol 2006; 60:489–498.
29. Ning N, Pan Q, Zheng F, et al. Cancer stem cell vaccination confers significant antitumor immunity. Cancer Res 2012; 72:1853–1864.

Chapter 3

PET-CT in head and neck cancer

Wai Lup Wong, Bal Sanghera, Peter Ross

INTRODUCTION

The aim of the chapter is to provide an overview of the current applications and emerging roles of positron emission tomography-computed tomography (PET-CT) in head and neck squamous cell carcinoma (HNSCC). Firstly, by way of background, a broad overview of the theoretical basis for PET-CT is considered. Then, a review of the generally accepted applications of 2-fluoro-2-deoxy-D-glucose (FDG) PET-CT in HNSCC is considered, followed by a discussion on the emerging role of FDG PET-CT. Next, the potential of PET radiotracers beyond FDG in HNSCC is highlighted. And finally, some observations regarding advances in PET-CT and in the broader context of current thinking regarding the adoption of new technology are discussed.

BACKGROUND

PET-CT is an imaging technique in which abnormalities of tissue metabolism are precisely superimposed onto anatomy. It relies on the premise that malignant cells are more metabolically active compared with nonmalignant cells. On this basis, a radiotracer which is radioactive analogue of a cellular molecule is given intravenously to the patient. It is taken up by cells. The cells recognise the analogue as 'foreign' and the radiotracer is trapped early in its metabolic pathway. Malignant cells trap more radiotracer compared with nonmalignant cells. Local radiotracer concentration can be measured in vivo. How? The unstable radiotracer decays by positron emission. Positrons travel a short distance in tissue before colliding with electrons. On collision, the annihilation reaction results in two photons known as gamma rays, each 511 kiloelectron volts (keV) emitted at approximately at 180% to each other. The photons are detected by opposing detectors. A computer reassembles these signals into images that represent radiotracer uptake in the part of the body scanned (**Figure 3.1 a** and **b**).

In addition to images of radiotracer uptake in tissue, with PET it is possible to obtain quantitative data and that being one of the main strengths of the technique. Direct measurement of radiotracer uptake is feasible. However, absolute quantification is

Wai Lup Wong BA [Hons] LLM FRCR FRCP, Mount Vernon Hospital, Northwood, UK. Email: wailupwong.wong@nhs.net (for correspondence)

Bal Sanghera PhD, Mount Vernon Hospital, Northwood, UK.

Peter Ross BSc BA [Hons] MSc, Department of Management, Birkbeck, University of London, London, UK.

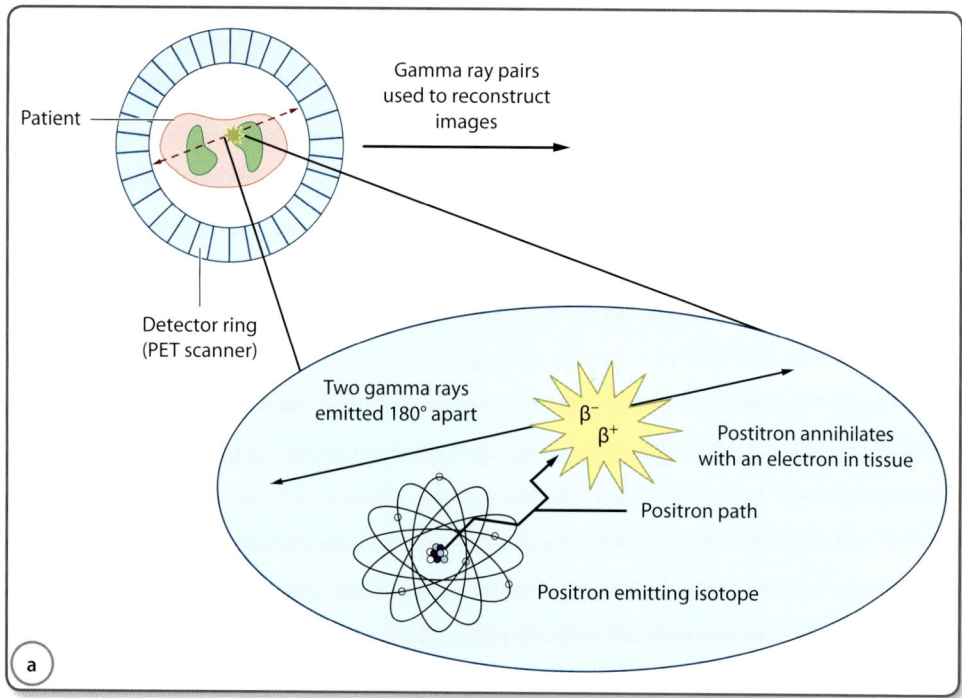

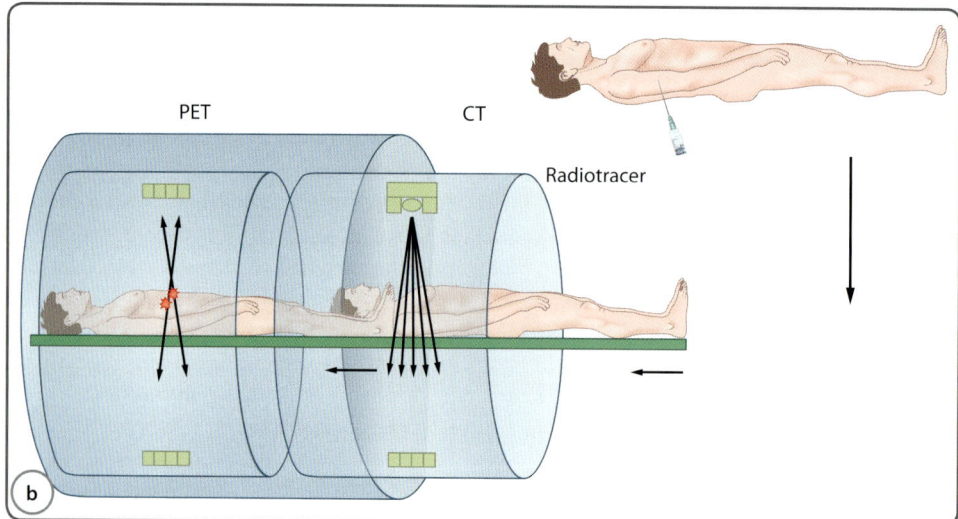

Figure 3.1 (a) The principles of positron emission tomography-computed tomography (PET-CT) imaging. Projection PET-CT shows a synchronous lung cancer in a patient who is being investigated for recurrent head and neck cancer. (b) Schematic representation of scanning with PET-CT. The patient is injected with the radiotracer. There is appropriate time interval before scanning to allow for radiotracer to be taken by abnormal tissue; in the case of FDG, a patient is usually scanned between 60 and 90 minutes following injection of 2-fluoro-2-deoxy-D-glucose (FDG). The patient then has a low-dose CT scan for attenuation correction and anatomical localisation of PET data. It is of diagnostic quality for detecting the majority of lung metastases. The PET scan follows. The radiation burden of one FDG PET-CT scan from vertex of skull vault to just below the pelvis is approximately equivalent to two whole body diagnostic CT scans.

usually only reserved for research studies because it is complicated to acquire and can require direct arterial blood sampling. Instead, standardised uptake value (SUV), and more specifically SUVmax of a lesion, is widely used in clinical practice. It provides an indirect and semiquantitative index of radiotracer uptake but with the advantage of being noninvasive. With regard to SUV, it is important to realise that there are many factors which influence SUV, including the time required to take the measurement post injection [1].

Depending on the radiotracer used, different aspects of tissue metabolism can be evaluated, including relative hypoxia and proliferative capacity of tissue. That said, the overwhelming majority of clinical studies use FDG which reflects glucose metabolism; cancer cells in general have higher glucose uptake compared with normal cells. FDG PET-CT has been used effectively for imaging a variety of malignancies including oesophageal, colorectal, lung cancer and lymphoma [2]. It has an established role in the assessment of patients with HNSCC.

INDICATIONS FOR FDG PET-CT IN HNSCC

A recent comparison of some of the main guidance on FDG PET-CT in HNSCC shows a high level of convergence between key evidence-based guidelines published on the use of FDG PET-CT in HNSCC [3]. Firstly, the authors found that there is almost universal recommendation for considering FDG PET-CT in occult primary patients and specifically before examination under anaesthesia. The approach is justified on grounds that it allows for targeted panendoscopy and avoids potential false positives if FDG PET-CT is done after biopsies. Secondly, there is general agreement on advocating FDG PET-CT for staging or restaging patients with high risk of disseminated disease including patients with advanced locoregional disease and patients harbouring primary sites which have a high propensity for disseminated disease such as nasopharyngeal cancer. Also, there is general agreement that FDG PET-CT should be considered in the investigation of lesions which remain indeterminate on usual assessment and where improved characterisation may change the treatment plan. And finally, there is consensus that there is inadequate data presently to recommend FDG PET-CT in the routine surveillance of asymptomatic patients with no clinical suspicion of disease.

It was highlighted in that commentary that there are two areas where guidelines are divided. Firstly, some guidelines including the Ontario guidelines do not include FDG PET-CT for diagnosing recurrence and for no clear reasons [4]. On the one hand, the Ontario panel acknowledged that there is compelling data supporting the use of FDG PET-CT in the diagnosis of recurrent cancer, especially if difficult to access and clinically examine sites, but on the other hand, the panel argued that the data are sparse. Agreed, there is a paucity of data on FDG PET-CT in the detection of recurrence, but dismissing the value of FDG PET-CT in this area ignores the weight of evidence that FDG PET is superior to conventional imaging for distinguishing treatment sequelae from recurrence [3]. There is no reason why PET-CT should lead to poorer results; on the contrary, there is evidence that PET-CT leads to more accurate results compared with FDG PET [5]. As the value of FDG PET in this area has already been compellingly proved, this is probably one explanation for the few PET-CT studies. Interestingly, but for reasons unclear, the Ontario panel included FDG PET-CT for investigation of nasopharyngeal carcinoma recurrence [4].

The other area where opinion is divided is in the use of PET-CT for residual disease assessment in patients with advanced neck disease following chemoradiotherapy. Some guidelines, including the National Comprehensive Cancer Network USA specifically

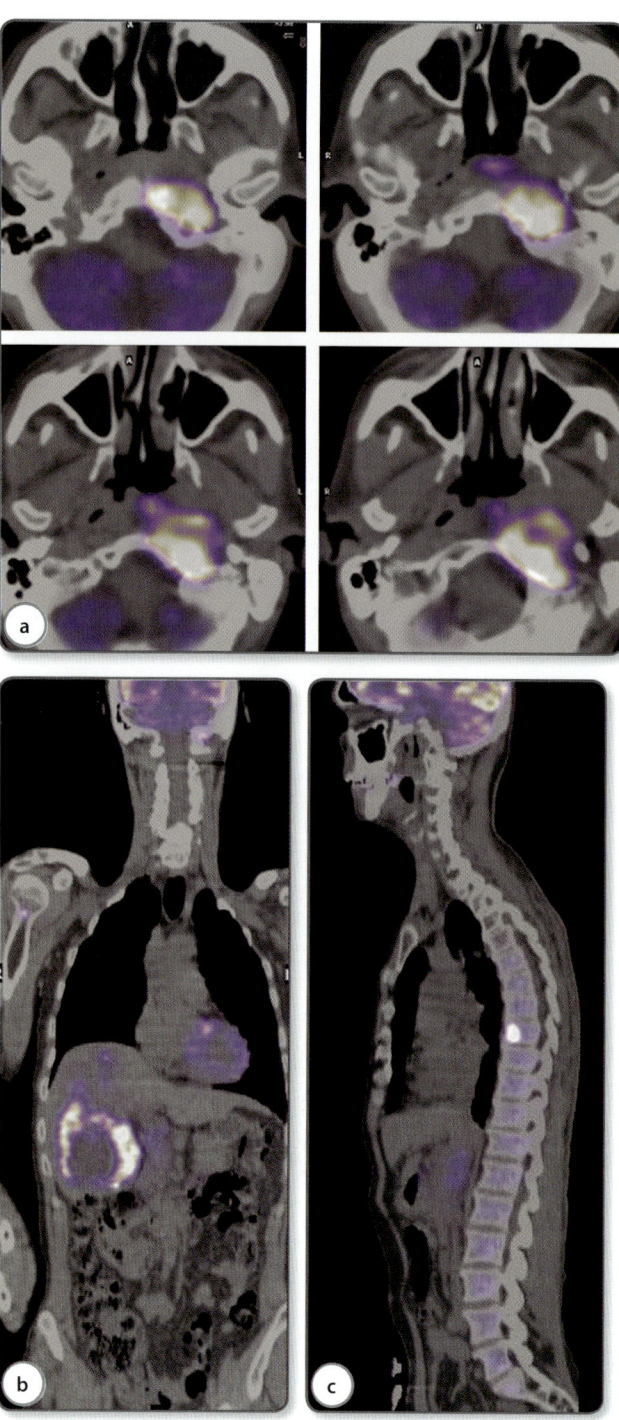

Figure 3.2 Patient with nasopharyngeal carcinoma. 2-Fluoro-2-deoxy-D-glucose positron emission tomography-computed tomography shows (a) the primary site, (b) the liver deposit and (c) radiotherapy humeral bone deposit in the midthoracic spine.

include this as an indication for FDG PET-CT, and other guidelines such as the Australia and New Zealand Association of Physicians in Nuclear Medicine Physicians (ANZAPNM) and Medicaid/Medicare are inclusive enough to include FDG PET-CT in this scenario [3]. However, others exclude it as an indication apparently due to lack of supportive evidence [3]. In the Ontario guidelines, two prospective studies were considered and they showed conflicting results. One study showed value and one showed no additional diagnostic advantage of FDG PET over CT [6,7]. Two points need to be made with regard to the study that showed no advantage. It was a PET and not a PET-CT study. The advantages of PET-CT over PET have been considered. FDG PET was done 7 weeks following completion of chemoradiotherapy. There is general consensus in the literature and clinically that misleading results occur when FDG PET is done before 8 weeks post-chemoradiotherapy [4]. Assessing the literature, FDG PET has a high negative predictive value in excess of 90% when done at least 8 weeks post-chemoradiotherapy [3]. Wang et al. showed that FDG PET had equally high accuracy in patients with clinically negative necks and patients with clinically apparent residual masses [9]. The UK guidelines are coy and add to the uncertainty [2]. They recommend FDG PET-CT for response assessment 3–6 months post-chemoradiotherapy in patients with residual masses. They remain silent regarding the neck with no residual mass. Forthcoming data from the nearly complete Health Technology Assessment PETNECK study funded by the Department of Health England will hopefully confirm the role of FDG PET-CT in this area.

EMERGING APPLICATIONS FOR FDG PET-CT

PET-CT-RT planning

FDG PET-CT is increasingly used for the delineation of radiotherapy therapy target volume, but not without some reservations. A recent review discusses the advantages and drawbacks afforded by using FDG PET-CT [9]. Benefits include a reduction in interobserver variability in gross tumour volume (GTV) delineation, reduction in size of the GTV and the identification of tumour that would not otherwise have been treated but for PET-CT, geographical misses. However, there is the major challenge of accurate delineation of tumour margins due to two main reasons: firstly, false-positive results due to inflammation may lead to overestimation of tumour margins; Secondly, when tumour margin delineation is dependant of functional imaging, there is at present no reliable method for determining the tumour margins and furthermore there is lack of a universally accepted and standardised method of identifying tumour margins. There are encouraging results of two studies where overall survival and event-free survival rates of patients treated with FDG PET-CT based intensity modulated radiotherapy (IMRT) were significantly better than for the control group. But, as Troost et al. highlighted these studies were small retrospective studies including heterogeneous patient populations, with short follow-up and using historical controls [10]. It is also not clear from the studies whether the improvements afforded in tumour control were due to PET-CT or due to other factors such as improved radiotherapy techniques [9]. So in this area more studies are needed to clarify the benefits of applying FDG PET-CT.

Early prediction of treatment response

In HNSCC, there has been recent revived enthusiasm for the use of induction chemotherapy. This is because of studies which showed that adding taxane, and specifically

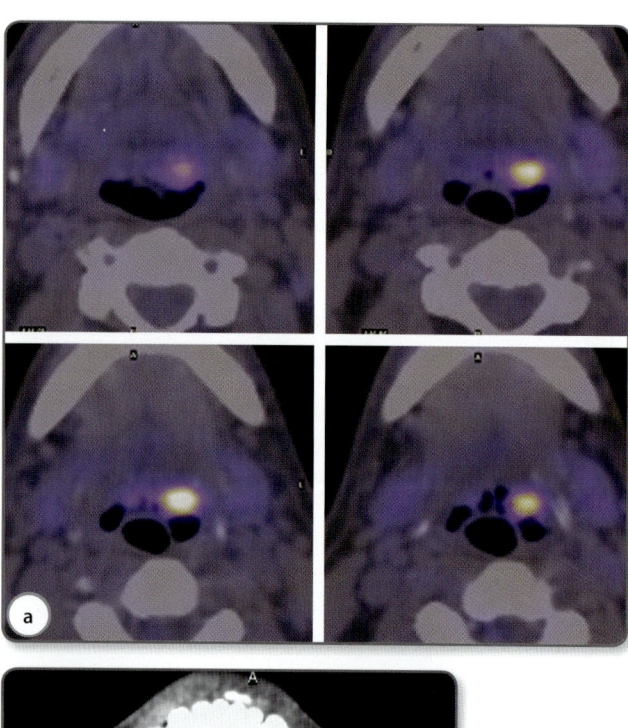

Figure 3.3 Patient presented with an enlarged node in the left level II of the neck. The node contained squamous cell carcinoma. No primary site was identified on usual assessment including flexible fibre optic nasoendoscopy, diagnostic computed tomography. (a) 2-Fluoro-2-deoxy-D-glucose positron emission tomography-computed tomography suggested a primary site in the lingual thyroid base of tongue, confirmed subsequently by EUA and biopsies. (b) The primary site was unclear even in retrospect on the diagnostic post intravenous contrast computed tomography.

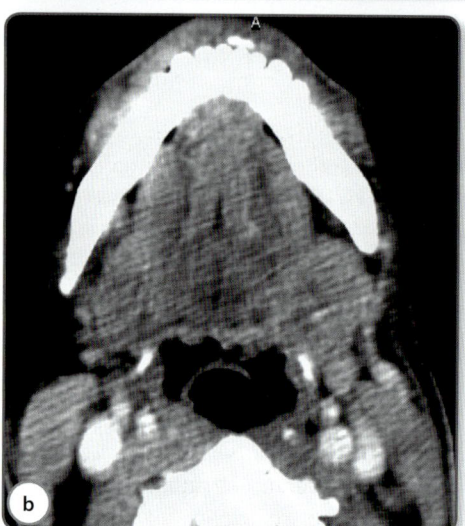

docetaxel and paclitaxel, to a chemotherapy regime of 5FU and cisplatinum results in significantly improved response rates compared with the combination of cisplatinum and 5-fluoro-uracil (5FU), and is cost-effective [10,11]. However, induction chemotherapy adds toxicity and prolongs treatment [12]. So, the ability to distinguish responders from nonresponders early during treatment would be ideal.

Notwithstanding that FDG PET-CT has been shown to be able to provide an early prediction in response to neoadjuvant chemotherapy in a variety of solid tumours including oesophageal carcinoma, there is currently only one published study where FDG PET-CT was used in conjunction with induction chemotherapy with docetaxcel, cisplatinum and 5FU prior to chemoradiotherapy, a small 15 patent pilot study. In that study, early therapeutic response on FDG PET-CT after two cycles of chemotherapy predicted event free survival. Of the 10 patients with a partial or complete response on FDG PET-CT, no patients relapsed during their follow-up period of between 3.8 and 25 months (median, 18.9 months). By contrast, four out of the five patients who showed no metabolic response had recurrences between 7.4 and 10.6 months. Metabolic response was defined as a decrease in SUVmax between the pretreatment FDG PET-CT and the FDG PET-CT after two cycles of chemotherapy [13].

PET RADIOTRACERS BEYOND FDG

FLT

Increased cellular proliferation is a feature malignant tissue which can be visualised and quantified on PET-CT with the thymidine analogue thymidine 3-deoxy-3-^{18}F-fluorothymidine (FLT). There is a direct correlation between FLT uptake and cell proliferation FLT and FLT provides an indirect marker of cell proliferation. The reason is as follows. During cell proliferation, there is increased DNA synthesis and there is a much higher thymidine kinase-1 (TK-1) activity than normal cells. FLT is taken up by cells and phosphorylated to monophosphate by TK-1. FLT monophosphate is not incorporated into DNA and is impermeable to the cell membrane Therefore, FLT monophosphate is metabolically trapped inside the cells and with proliferating cells trapping up to tenfold more FLT monophosphate compared with nonproliferating cells. So, FLT provides an index of cellular proliferation [15].

The role of FLT in the evaluation of HNSCC is unsettled. There does not appear definite advantage of FLT over FDG for staging HNSCC. With regard to the primary site, several small pilot studies showed FLT has similar sensitivity to FDG for detecting HNSCC, but the uptake of FLT was lower compared with FDG; these results were observed in similar studies with other malignant tumours [14]. Notwithstanding this observation, if it is because FLT is only taken up by malignant cells and FDG malignant and benign cells, and this has yet to be resolved, then this may be of value of more precisely delineating extent of primary site in the rare occasion when this is important for the treatment planning. With regard to nodal disease, FLT is of limited value as both malignant and reactive nodes show uptake and FLT cannot replace elective treatment of the neck [15]. FLT is of limited value for detecting metastases [16]. The superiority of FLT over FDG for characterising lung lesion, the common site of distant metastases, is unclear. Bone and liver metastases will not easily be detected as there is normal intense uptake of FLT by these organs.

Where FLT may have a role is for detecting residual disease following radiotherapy (RT) and chemotherapy and to predict outcome of radiotherapy and chemoradiotherapy treatment. A decrease in FLT uptake in HNSCC occurs as early as 2 weeks into treatment, and FLT response during treatment may accurately predict locoregional disease control. Troost et al. showed, in 10 patients with oropharyngeal cancer undergoing concomitant chemoradiotherapy and IMRT, that there was significant FLT decrease in the primary site and neck nodes between pretherapy scan and a scan as early as 2 weeks after start of treatment which preceded morphological changes [17]. In one prospective study of 48 patients treated with RT and concomitant chemoradiotherapy, decreased FLT uptake in the second week of treatment and in the fourth treatment week was associated with better 3 years disease-free survival [18]. In study of 28 patients treated with concomitant chemoradiotherapy, FLT PET-CT 5 weeks after the end of treatment more accurately predicted 3 years control of disease at the primary site and in the post-treatment neck compared with an FDG at the same point in time [19].

Radiotracers for detecting hypoxia

Tumours, including 1–2 mm tumours, require a new blood supply to survive. Angiogenesis occurs. But these blood vessels are very tortuous and leaky leading to inefficient oxygenation of the tumour and resulting in hypoxic cells. Hypoxic cells are radioresistant requiring three times as much radiation to kill them in compared with cells that are not hypoxic. Delivering a dose of radiotherapy to the whole tumour which is effective for the killing of the hypoxic cells is not possible because of the damage it will cause to surrounding normal tissue. Imaging of hypoxia would provide the opportunity to apply radiotherapy to the subvolume of hypoxic cells only.

PET tracers for detecting hypoxia include two main groups. One formed by the fluorinated nitroimidazole compounds include 1-[2-nitro-1-imidazolyl-3[^{18}-F] fluoro-2-propanol ([^{18}F]FMISO), 1-(5-[^{18}F]fluoro-5-deoxy-α-D-arabinofuranosyl)-2-nitro-imidazole ([^{18}F] FAZA), ^{18}F-2-(2-nitro-imidazol-1-yl)-N-(3,3,3-trifluropropyl)-acetamide (^{18}F-EF3) and ^{18}F-fluoroerythronitromidazole (^{18}F-FETNIM). The other class is copper isotopes of varying half-life, including ^{60}Cu with a half-life of 23.7 minutes; ^{61}Cu 3.3 hours, ^{62}Cu 9.74 minutes, ^{62}Cu 12.7 hours, and labelled to copper-diacetyl-bis(N^4-methylthiosemicabazone) (Cu-ATSM) and copper-pyruvaldehyde-bis(N^4-methylthiosemicarbazone (Cu-PTSM). There is as yet no one clear front runner. MISO is the most commonly used and best validated tracer for hypoxia imaging, and most studies have shown correlation between hypoxia and MISO uptake [20]. But it is only slowly cleared from the blood compartment, and the radiotracer passively diffuses into the cell which takes a relatively long time. This means that for imaging to be effective it has to be done between 2 and 3 hours post injection [21]. There is as yet inadequate data to recommend the other tracers as superior.

11C-choline PET-CT

^{11}C-choline PET-CT, in a pilot study, was of value in the assessment of patients with nasopharyngeal carcinoma. ^{11}C-choline improved the delineation of orbital and skull involvement compared with FDG PET-CT [22]. Because there is intense FDG uptake in normal brain and extraocular eye muscles, physiological uptake of ^{11}C-choline in brain and extraocular eye muscles is minimal. The advantage of ^{11}C-coline beyond this specific scenario has been questioned [23].

SOME BROADER OBSERVATIONS

When considering the adoption of new technologies such as new clinical guidelines and emerging radiotracers, it is important to remember the broader context within which they are situated. Traditionally, medical research adopts an approach based on objective rationality. This is evident in the way scientific research is usually depersonalised so as to lend 'objectivity' and consistency' to research findings. However, critiques of this approach argue it fails to take account of the complexities attached to the process of data interpretation. Nonprogrammed decision making, i.e. decisions made in complex and unfamiliar areas where there are no precedents, such as those related to topics that are complex with problematic definitions, where information is unavailable and solutions are difficult to identify, is rarely made with perfect rationality and that probably includes consensus guideline generation [24-26]. Factors beyond robustness of data often influence decision making in guidelines [27]. These include the opinions, clinical experience and composition of the guideline development group, as well as health care budgets. What is needed is not only an awareness but also the development of the vocabulary to narrate the decision-making process.

To support understanding in this area, cognitive organisation theorists like Karl Weick have developed models of organisations as interpretation systems that take account of the processes adopted by organisations when interpreting the data. Weick's enactment model conceptualises the interpretation process into three stages: (1) scanning of the environment for evidence (2) interpretation of evidence and (3) action, e.g. development of clinical guidelines [28]. Building on the idea that knowledge is a social construction of collective sense making, the model implies that decision makers enact the environment they anticipate. Such an approach can further our understanding of decision making, by making us aware of two key social influences. Firstly, the decision maker's beliefs about the analysability of the data and secondly the extent to which the decision-making body is passive as opposed to proactive in seeking out corroborating data. In other words, if decision makers view the evidence as ambiguous, judgement, intuition and subjective normative factors will play a larger role in the interpretation process. Equally where one decision-making body is more passive in comparison to another in seeking out answers, the interpretation will quite likely be different. Applied to considerations surrounding radiotracer or guideline effectiveness, the theory tells us that effectiveness cannot be separated from the decision maker's perceptions. This is because decision makers will always respond to their perceptions and enact the environment they anticipate by constructing an interpretation that seems reasonable.

Awareness of the role of subjective factors and the capacity for decision makers to enact their perception of the environment have changed the way in which many organisations now analyse their markets. For example, when organisations undertake analysis of future pharmaceutical applications, it is often not limited to a purely rational analysis of objective market conditions and trends but may also involve a process of equivocality and narrative creation whereby key decision makers are asked to contribute their perception of the future [29].

So what are the possible implications beyond academic interest if evaluating evidence is a less than a precise science? Firstly, evidence needs to be viewed as open to more than one interpretation. If facts speak for themselves, this may only be because observers happen to be saying the same things. Secondly, decision makers need to be aware of the assumptions they unwittingly bring to collective discussions. Thirdly, rather than amassing evidence, decision makers may also need to guide interpretation by providing a vision for the future. In this way, we acknowledge the bounded nature of rationality of decision making. In the final analysis, how evidence is evaluated and acted on is influenced by the assumptions people hold and the visions people believe in. Such a view, with its different emphasis on what is important, can expand our understanding of decision processes and implies a different set of prescriptions for managers and practitioners [30].

Key points for clinical practice

- Positron emission tomography-computed tomography (PET-CT), an imaging technique in tissue metabolism, is precisely localised onto anatomy and relies on the premise that malignant cells ate more metabolically active compared with nonmalignant cells.

- 2-Fluoro-2-deoxy-D-glucose (FDG) is the most widely used PET-CT radiotracer in clinical practice.

- There is almost universal recommendation for considering the use of FDG PET-CT in patients with occult head and neck primary, and specifically before examination under anaesthesia (EUA).

- There is general agreement on advocating FDG-PET-CT for staging and restaging patients with a high risk of disseminated disease.

- There is general consensus that FDG PET-CT should be considered in the investigation of lesions which remain indeterminate on usual assessment and where improved characterisation may change treatment plan.

- There remains uncertainty of the precise role for FDG PET-CT in the assessment of residual disease in patients with advanced neck nodal disease following chemoradiotherapy, in the assessment of patients with suspected recurrent disease, planning radiotherapy treatment and in the assessment of early response to induction and neoadjuvant treatment.

- PET radiotracers beyond FDG which are of current interest for the assessment of head and neck squamous cell carcinoma include thymidine 3-deoxy-3-18F-flurotymidine, radiotracers for detecting hypoxia and 11C-choline

- Decision making is rarely made with perfect rationality; how evidence is evaluated and acted on is influenced by the assumptions people hold and the visions people believe in.

REFERENCES

1. Kwee TC Cheng G, Lam MGEH. SUVmax of 2.5 should not be embraced as a magic threshold for separating benign from malignant lesions. EJNMMI 2013; 40:1475.
2. PP Hsu, Sabitini DM. Cancer cell metabolism: Warburg and beyond. Cell 2008; 134:703.
3. Barrington S, Scarsbrook A. Evidence based Indications for the use of PET/CT in the UK 2012. London: Royal College of Physicians and Royal College of Radiologists, 2012.
4. Wong WL, Ross P, Corcoran M. Evidence based guidelines recommendations on the use of PET CT imaging in head and neck cancer from Ontario and guidelines in general – some observations. Clin Oncol 2013; 25:242–245.
5. Yoo J, Henderson S, Walker-Dyke C. Evidence-based guideline recommendations on the use of positron emission tomography in head and neck cancer. Clin Oncol 2013; 25:e33.
6. Schroder H, Yeung HWD, Gonen M, Kraus D, Larson SM. Head and neck : clinical usefulness and accuracy of PET CT image fusion. Radiology 2004; 231:65.
7. Porceddu SV, Jarmolowski E, Hicks RJ, et al. Utility of PET for the detection of disease in residual neck nodes after [chemo] radiotherapy in head and neck cancer. Head Neck 2005; 27:175.
9. Wang Y-F, Liu R-S, Chu P-Y, et al. PET in surveillance of head and neck squamous cell carcinoma after definitive chemoradiotherapy. Head Neck 2009; 31:442.
10. Troost GC, Schinagl DAX, Bussink J, Oyen WMJ, Kaanders JHAM. Clinical evidence on PET CT for radiation therapy planning in head and neck tumours. Radiother Oncol 2010; 96:328–334.
11. Blanchard P, Bourhis J, Lacas B, et al. Taxane-cisplatin-fluorouracil as induction chemotherapy in locally advanced head and neck cancers: an individual patient data meta-analysis of the meta-analysis of chemotherapy in head and neck cancer group. Meta-Analysis of Chemotherapy in Head and Neck Cancer, Induction Project, Collaborative Group. J Clin Oncol 2013; 31:2854–2860.

12. Adelstein DJ. Induction redux: once more with taxanes. J Clin Oncol 2005; 23:8556.
13. Abgal R, Le Roux P-Y, Keromnes N, et al. Early prediction of survival following induction chemotherapy with DCF using FDG PET/CT imaging in patients with locally advanced head and neck cancer. Eur J Nucl Med Mol Imaging 2012; 39:1839–1847.
14. Hoshikawa H, Nishiyama Y, Kishino T, et al. Comparison of FLT-PET and FDG-PET for visualization of head and neck squamous cell cancers. Mol Imaging Biol 2011; 13:1172–1177.
15. Troost EG, Vogel WV, Merkx MA, et al. 18F-FLT PET does not discriminate between reactive and metastatic lymph nodes in primary head and neck cancer patients. J Nucl 2007; 48:726–735.
16. Hoshikawa H, Kishino T, Mori T, et al. The value of 18F-FLT for detecting second primary cancers and distant metastases in head and neck cancer. Clin Nucl Med 2013; 38:318–324.
17. Troost EG, Bussink J, Hoffmann AL, et al. 18F-FLT PET/CT for early response monitoring and dose escalation in oropharyngeal tumors. J Nucl Med 2010; 51:866–874.
18. Hoeben BA, Troost EG, Span PN, et al. 18F-FLT PET during radiotherapy or chemoradiotherapy in head and neck squamous cell carcinoma is an early predictor of outcome. J Nucl Med 2013; 54:532–540.
19. Kishino T, Hoshikawa H, Nishiyama Y, Yamamoto Y, Mori N. Usefulness of 3'-deoxy-3'-18F-fluorothymidine PET for predicting early response to chemoradiotherapy in head and neck cancer. J Nucl Med 2012; 53:1521–1527.
20. Horsman MR, Motensen LS, Peterson, Busk M, Overgaard J. Imaging hypoxia to improve RT outcomes. Nat Rev Clin Oncol 2012; 9:674–687.
21. Carlin S, Humm JL. PET of hypoxia: current and future perspectives. JNM 2012; 53:1171.
22. Wu HB, Wang QS, Wang MF, et al. Preliminary study of 11C-choline PET/CT for T staging of locally advanced nasopharyngeal carcinoma: comparison with 18F-FDGH PET/CT. J Nucl Med 2011; 52:341–346.
23. Ito K, Kubota K, Morooka M, Yokoyama J. Comparison of PET CT with F18-FDG and with C11-choline for the detection of recurrence of head and neck cancer after radiotherapy. J Nucl Med 2009; 50:1780.
24. Simon HA. Administrative behavior. New York: McMillan; 1947.
25. Simon HA. The new science of management decisions. New York: Harper & Row; 1960.
26. Miller SJ, Wilson DC. Perspectives on organized decision making. In: Clegg SR, Hardy C, Lawrence TB, Nord WR (eds.), The handbook of organisation studies, 2nd edn. London: Sage; 2006:469–484.
27. Woolf SH, Grol R, Hutchinson A, Eccles M, Grimshaw J. Potential benefits, limitations and harms of clinical guidelines. Br Med J 1999; 318:527.
28. Daft R, Weick K. Towards a model of organizations as interpretation systems. Acad Manag Rev 1984; 9:282–289.
29. Hatch MJ, Cuncliffe AL (eds). Organization theory, modern symbolic and postmodern perspectives. Oxford: Oxford University Press; 2013.
30. Smircich L, Stubbart C. Strategic management in an enacted world. [1985] Academy of Management Review 10:724-736

Chapter 4

Middle ear implants

HISTORICAL ASPECTS

Whilst early attempts of active middle ear implants go back to the 1930 of the last century, the current motivation for the development of middle ear implant systems should consider the context of hearing aids and other implantable hearing systems.

In the early times of hearing aids, there was a limited ability to offer the patient sufficient energy to reach a proper gain to improve the understanding of speech. Therefore, active middle ear implants were in the 90s assumed to close the audiological gap between cochlear implants (CIs) and hearing aids. The disadvantage of ear moulds which close the external auditory canal and potentially cause eczema, chronic otitis externa should be overcome by active middle ear systems, which allowed the external auditory canal to remain open. This was a great advantage in terms of clinical indications [1]. The problem of limited functional gain obtained by hearing aids in the high-frequency range seemed to be resolved by active middle ear implants.

On one hand, current developments of hearing aids with modern high-frequency algorithms (sound recovery, frequency transposition) and expanding indication criteria for CIs by excellent results in patients with residual hearing limit the group of patients with classical audiological indications. On the other hand, recent developments of extended audiological indication criteria for those with conductive or mixed hearing loss originating from 'alternative coupling' of actors (e.g. to ossicle residues) the round/oval window (RW/OW) or third window will include new patient groups, which were the domain of bone – anchored hearing systems or hearing aids so far. Choosing the right hearing system is – in a fast developing and changing field of hearing systems, overlapping indications and country-specific economic limitations – a demanding task.

PRINCIPLES

With the exception of anomalies, active middle ear implants are a second-line treatment option. Before deciding for an active middle ear implant, modern hearing aids have to be sufficiently tried. Before choosing an active middle ear system in cases of conductive or mixed hearing loss, additional middle ear surgeries should have made the outer ear canal dry and ready to use hearing aids.

Ingo Todt MD, Associate Professor, Department of Otolaryngology, Head and Neck Surgery, Unfallkrankenhaus, Berlin, Germany. E-mail: todt@gmx.net (for correspondence)

INDICATIONS AND DIFFERENTIAL INDICATIONS

Currently, we can differentiate between an audiological and a clinical indication for middle ear implant systems. The middle ear implant systems should be taken into consideration if other less invasive systems do not cover the audiological indication criteria to provide an acceptable speech understanding. The audiological indication for a 'classical' incus coupling of the Vibrant Soundbridge (VSB) as given by the manufacturer can be seen in **Figure 4.1**. The one for the middle ear transducer (MET) is described in **Figure 4.2**.

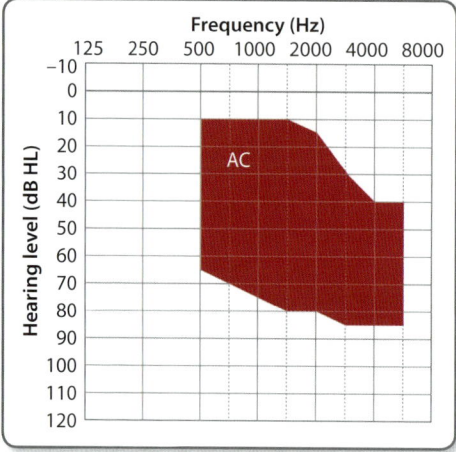

Figure 4.1 Audiological indication criteria for the Vibrant Soundbridge and pure sensorineural hearing loss.

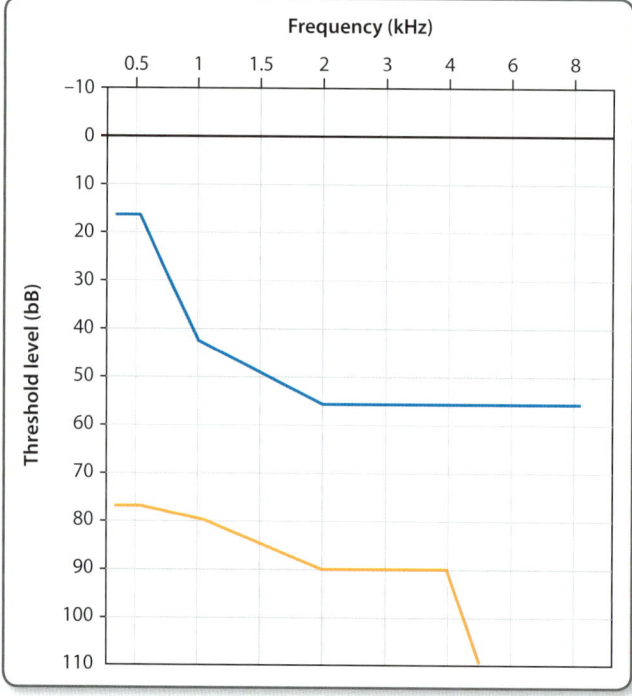

Figure 4.2 Audiological indication criteria for the middle ear transducer and pure sensorineural hearing loss.

The audiological indication criteria for a conductive and mixed hearing loss for the VSB are given in **Figure 4.3**. Since the development of other, competing hearing systems is fast ongoing, a permanent comparison of the indications of the different systems should be attempted.

Looking at the pure sensorineural hearing loss (SNHL) indication, hearing aid systems with frequency compression or transposition algorithms are trying to cover the audiological indication field of high-frequency SNHL or 'ski-slope' hearing loss (Phonak Sound Recovery, Widek Frequency Transposition) which is overlapping with the recommended indication for the VSB. Therefore, a sufficient testing period (minimum 2 weeks) of current hearing aids should be preferred in those cases. Since the indication corridor for the MET covers even more the low-frequency range, other specific power hearing aids should be tested prior to surgery.

If the hearing loss exceeds 60–70 dB, an overlap with CI systems can occur (e.g. a hybrid or electric and acoustic stimulation). Looking at those pure conductive hearing losses, a fitting with a bone conductive system should be kept in mind. The transcutaneous systems (BAHA, Cochlear, Sydney, Australia; Ponto, Oticon, Denmark) and even the percutaneous systems (Vibrant Bonebridge, Medel, Innsbruck, Austria) offer in some cases a better solution for the patient (i.e. less risky) than the active middle ear implants. However, those bone conductive systems have only the audiological ability to close an air-bone gap. This limits their indication corridor to cases of <35 dB bone conduction (BC) SNHL. Additionally, a time and disease-related progressive threshold shift can be seen and should be kept in mind.

Looking at combined hearing losses on average, hearing aids can overcome an air-bone gap of 30–35 dB. In cases of larger air-bone gaps (ABGs), a middle ear implant can be indicated. In general, even in those cases a hearing aid should be tested before the possible implantation of an active middle ear system. Although a medical indication cannot be completely separated from the audiological indication, there are specific constellations where an active middle ear systems is the only medical solution for a patient.

In cases of chronic otitis externa in combination with a SNHL after multiple tests with ear moulds, only an active middle ear system can help the patient. Hearing losses in cases of radical cavities ('canal- wall- down') caused by cholesteatoma surgeries can often only be treated by an active middle ear system since fitting with hearing aids leads in many cases to an otorrhoea.

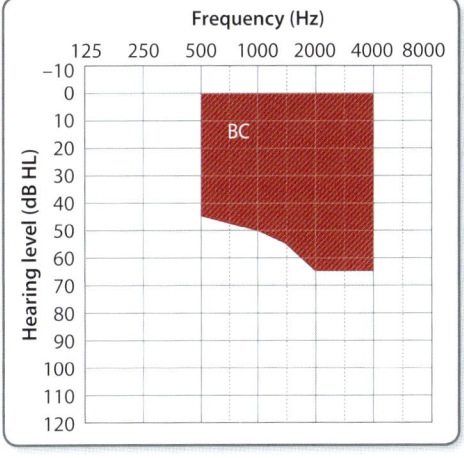

Figure 4.3 Audiological indication criteria for the Vibrant Soundbridge for the inner ear function in cases of mixed hearing loss.

Anomalies especially in children are described to be treated by active middle ear systems, but in those cases a critical comparison with bone conductive systems should be done. Although described as a one-step treatment in cases of otosclerosis, the indication for an active middle ear implant system should be critically considered. A regular indication for an active middle ear implant system is an ear with chronic otitis media, which, after multiple middle ear surgeries, has become dry, but with persisting mixed hearing loss.

SYSTEMS

There are currently five different middle ear systems on the European market. The VSB system (Medel, Austria, Innsbruck) consists of an implanted receiver with a magnet, demodulator and a cable attached to an electromagnetic actor called floating mass transducer (FMT). This actor has an attached clip, which allows the fixation to the long process of the incus. The FMT can be fixed to the stapes head or after removal of the clip attached to the RW. The addition of coupler elements offers a standardised attachment to the RW, the OW or the stapes suprastructure.

The audioprocessor is in the fifth generation and has a 16 canal processor and two directional microphones. The system has a conformity marking of the European community market (CE) and is currently FDA approved for an incus attachment application. The MET systems (Boulder, Colorado, USA) consist of an implant with a magnet and a spoil with an electromagnetically driven actor which is attached to the head of the incus, the RW or to the stapes head. The system is fixed in the mastoid cavity by a plating system. The system has a CE mark. The Carina system consists of the same ossicular actor and fixation system in the mastoid. In contrast to the MET, a fully implantable microphone and a reloadable battery are attached. The system has a CE mark.

The direct acoustic cochlear stimulation (DACS) system consists of a magnet and a receiver. The receiver is fixed in the mastoid cavity by a plating system. The actor is electromagnetically driven. The actor contains a rod with an element for the fixation for a stapes prosthesis. The audioprocessor is the known cochlear freedom audioprocessor with specific modifications. The system has recently reached the CE mark.

The Esteem system (Envoy Medical, St. Paul, Minnesota, USA) is a fully implantable system and consists of a magnet and a receiver. A sensor which is attached to the malleolus catches the natural sound and transmits the signal to the receiver, which converts the signals and sends them to a piezo actor which is connected to the stapes. The ossicular chain has to be interrupted to prevent feedback. The system is FDA approved and has the CE mark.

The Maxum system (Ototronix, Texas, USA) is similar to the previously known Soundtec system. It consists of a stapes joint attached magnet and a specific ear canal device. The ear canal device steers the magnet by the application of a magnetic field. The device has the FDA approval and the CE mark.

SURGERIES

The different systems follow – with the exception of the Maxum system – a transmastoidal route for implantation. The usual surgical approach for the attachment of the VSB system at the long process of the incus consists of a mastoidectomy and a posterior tympanotomy. The FMT-clip is pushed onto the incus and crimped. Additional fixation to minimise surgical variations in the quality of attachment has been performed by the addition of bone cement or the push over of a Soft-Clip stapes prosthesis head. Surgical approaches without a mastoidectomy, but burying a canal through the external auditory canal, have been described.

In cases of pure conductive or mixed hearing loss, the FMT can be attached to different structures. Besides, the previously described surgical approach via a posterior tympanotomy can be performed in cases of canal-wall-down surgeries. For those cases, a two-step procedure consisting of a partial obliteration with cartilage, Palva flap, bone pate... and secondly a FMT attachment is recommended. In this way, the risk of a cable extrusion is minimised, and in addition, a revision without risking the implant is possible.

The attachment to the RW was performed for the first time by Colletti [2] in 2005. The RW attachment has been described in different ways. Whilst a cartilage support behind the FMT is commonly used, the contact between RW and FMT can vary. Whilst Colletti used Tutopatch, others place the FMT directly on the RW. Alternatively fascia, cartilage, Ivalon or a Kurz (Dusslingen, Germany) coupler is used. Common sense is that the RW should be well visualised after removal of the promontorial lip before placing the FMT. The frequently found differences in diameter between RW and the FMT have to be considered.

If persisting, an attachment on the stapes can be performed by a direct crimping of the FMT-clip onto it. The introduction of Kurz couplers (Clip, Bell, OW) allowed a more standardised attachment of the FMT to middle ear structures. The attachment on the OW has been described by the positioning of a cartilage piece with perichondrium on the footplate and wrapping it around the FMT. Newer developments allow the attachment on the OW with a specific total ossicular replacement prosthesis (TORP)-like coupler. The coupler is stabilised in the OW niche with a cartilage shoe [3].

A general recommendation for a coupling site of the FMT cannot be given. Since the audiological aim of an aided hearing threshold at 25–35 dB can be reached with all kinds of coupling, the chosen coupling site depends on the anatomic situation, the experience and preference of the surgeon and can easily be modified throughout surgery. In cases of occluded RW, high jugular bulb and fixed OW, the burring of an artificial third window and the attachment of the FMT directly on the endosteum has been described.

Even the fixation of the FMT additional to a stapes prosthesis on the long process of the incus called 'Power-Stapes' is known. Alternatively to stapes surgery, the direct insertion of a specific FMT coupler in a stapedotomy hole was successfully performed [4].

The MET surgery consists of a mastoidectomy. Mastoid size needs to be confirmed preoperatively to verify a proper ability to place the plating system for the actor inside the cavity and to exclude a low middle fossa obliterating the access to the short process of the incus. The actor and its transmission rod are attached to the incus for cases of SNHL. The actors load on the short process of the incus needs to be determined. In cases of conductive or mixed hearing loss, the coupling element of the actor can be positioned through a posterior tympanotomy on the RW with added fascia or with a specific coupling element on the stapes head [5]. A solution in cases of nonpersisting external canal wall is so far to our knowledge not described. In cases of Carina surgeries, the position of the microphone needs to be considered. It is recommended to be placed the microphone not under the temporalis muscle to minimise secondary noise by chewing.

The DACS systems actor position is even determined by a plating system. The actor is directed through a posterior tympanotomy over the OW. After a stapedotomy, a stapes prosthesis is inserted and fixed on the specific rod element of the actor. The vibration of the actor drives the stapes prosthesis. So far the indication of the system is limited to stapes surgery cases.

The Esteem surgery consists of a mastoidectomy and a very exact laser Doppler vibrometric controlled positioning of the sensor and the actor on the malleolus and the stapes head. The Maxum surgery can be performed, in contrast to the previous surgeries, in local anaesthesia. The surgery consists of a regular elevation of the tympanic membrane followed by an opening of the incudostapedial joint. Then the magnet is placed through the joint and the joint is closed. Disadvantage is a mandatory device in the ear canal.

RESULTS

The published results of the different systems depend very much on the included number of patients and the specific audiologic criteria. Therefore, a direct comparison of the systems is difficult to achieve.

The audiological result with the VSB system in cases of pure SNHL described a functional gain (aided hearing threshold over BC) of up to 30 dB [6]. The hearing gain (aided hearing threshold over AC) in cases of pure conductive and mixed hearing loss is described to be between 30 and 65 dB [3]. A difference between the different coupling options at the stapes showed no significant advantage of one over another [7]. All applications offer a sufficient gain to reach the target hearing threshold of 25–35 dB.

This holds true for all systems. The MET systems data described a functional gain between 15–20 and 39 dB [8,9]. The DACS system offers a functional gain of 17 dB and a hearing gain of 46 dB [10]. Data of the Esteem system showed a functional gain of 12 dB [11]. Maxum data showed a functional gain of 26 dB [12]. A subjective advantage in comparison to conventional hearing aids with its ear moulds has been described for all systems.

SPECIAL CONSIDERATIONS

The MRI compatibility of active middle ear implants is an important topic nowadays since the number of scans/lifetime is rising, as well as the number of implants and the tesla magnetic strength. Although only for the VSB system and the Maxum/Soundtec system described, a defined 'magnet shadow' (i.e. blackening) artefact was reported for both [13,14] and can be assumed for all systems.

Complications due to MRI scanning were described, but without serious medical complications (pain, dislocation of FMT) reported for the VSB at 1.5 T. Hearing losses or dislocations of the ossicular chain were not found when systematically investigating this subject [15]. The Maxum system is approved for 0.3 T scans [14], but no experiences exist beyond this limit.

Key points for clinical practice

- The number of patients who are candidates for active middle ear implants is highly limited in SNHL [16]. Those patients with mixed hearing loss are considered as the main patient population to be supplied with active middle ear implants.
- The treatment with active middle ear implants is a second-line treatment with the exception of anomalies.
- A trial with modern digital hearing aids is mandatory.

REFERENCES

1. Lenarz T, Weber BP, Mack KF, Battmer RD, Gnadeberg D. The Vibrant Soundbridge System: a new kind of hearing aid for sensorineural hearing loss. 1: function and initial clinical experiences. Laryngorhinootologie 1998; 77:247–255.
2. Colletti V, Soli SD, Carner M, Colletti L. Treatment of mixed hearing losses via implantation of a vibratory transducer on the round window. Int J Audiol 2006; 45(10):600-608.
3. Luers JC, Hüttenbrink KB, Zahnert T, Bornitz M, Beutner D. Vibroplasty for mixed and conductive hearing loss. Otol Neurotol 2013; 34:1005–1012.
4. Arauz SL, Mercandino EC, Campo E, Arauz SA. Vibrant Soundbridge-ubucacion en ventana oval utilizando proteseis-ad hoc. Otorinolaringologica 2007; 4:10–15.
5. Martin C, Deveze A, Richard C, et al. European results with totally implantable carina placed on the round window: 2-year follow-up. Otol Neurotol 2009; 30:1196–1203.
6. Todt I, Seidl RO, Ernst A. Hearing benefit of patients after Vibrant Soundbridge implantation. ORL J Otorhinolaryngol Relat Spec 2005; 67:203–206.
7. Coordes A, Ernst A, Todt I. Assessment of VSB attachments for the stapes head coupling. Int CI, Baltimore,3-5 May 2012, Abstract #237802.
8. Jenkins HA, Niparko JK, Slattery WH, Neely JG, Fredrickson JM. Otologics Middle Ear Transducer Ossicular Stimulator: performance results with varying degrees of sensorineural hearing loss. Acta Otolaryngol. 2004; 124:391–394.
9. Tringali S, Perrot X, Berger P, et al. Otologics middle ear transducer with contralateral conventional hearing aid in severe sensorineural hearing loss: evolution during the first 24 months. Otol Neurotol 2010; 31:630–636.
10. Lenarz T, Zwartenkot JW, Stieger C, et al. Multicenter study with a direct acoustic cochlear implant. Otol Neurotol 2013; 34:1215–1225.
11. Chen DA, Backous DD, Arriaga MA, et al. Phase 1 clinical trial results of the Envoy System: a totally implantable middle ear device for sensorineural hearing loss. Otolaryngol Head Neck Surg 2004; 131:904–916.
12. Silverstein H, Atkins J, Thompson JH Jr, Gilman N. Experience with the SOUNDTEC implantable hearing aid. Otol Neurotol 2005; 26:211–217.
13. Todt I, Seidl RO, Mutze S, Ernst A. MRI scanning and incus fixation in vibrant soundbridge implantation. Otol Neurotol 2004; 25:969–972.
14. Dyer RK Jr, Nakmali D, Dormer KJ. Magnetic resonance imaging compatibility and safety of the SOUNDTEC Direct System. Laryngoscope 2006; 116:1321–1333.
15. Todt I, Wagner J, Goetze R, et al. MRI scanning in patients implanted with a Vibrant Soundbridge. Laryngoscope 2011; 121:1532.
16. Junker R, Gross M, Todt I, Ernst A. Functional gain of already implanted hearing devices in patients with sensorineural hearing loss of varied origin and extent: Berlin experience. Otol Neurotol 2002; 23:452–456.

Chapter 5

Tissue hypoxia in chronic otitis media

Mahmood F Bhutta, Michael T Cheeseman

INTRODUCTION

Middle ear surgery is predominantly indicated for the treatment or prevention of the consequences of chronic otitis media (OM), whether that is persistent middle ear effusion, or tympanic erosion resulting from retraction pockets or cholesteatoma.

Clinically, the archetypal form of chronic otitis media is chronic otitis media with effusion (COME) otherwise known as 'glue ear,' where an effusion occupying the middle ear cleft may cause hearing loss. The pathological correlate of COME is an upregulation of the number and activity of goblet cells in the tympanic mucosa, leading to a persistent secretory effusion [1]. Epidemiological studies indicate that glue ear is a risk factor for squamous middle ear disease: patients developing either tympanic membrane retraction or cholesteatoma often have a preceding history of COME [2–5], although the biological mechanisms linking these disease entities are still a matter of debate.

Acute otitis media (AOM) is prevalent chiefly in childhood and is due to the ascent of resident nasopharyngeal bacterial flora into the middle ear, almost invariably preceded by a viral upper respiratory tract infection. AOM typically results in a middle ear effusion that is initially purulent, then becomes mucoid or serous, and then eventually resolves.

In a population of children with AOM, the time taken for an individual to resolve of effusion is variable, and is well modelled by an exponential decay function (**Figure 5.1**) [1]. In this epidemiological model, most children with middle ear effusion will eventually improve, but as the curve approaches the asymptote, there are a small proportion of children with persistent effusion, and a smaller proportion still in whom effusion persists into adulthood, and often then for the rest of their life.

Although in many cases AOM appears to be the trigger of COME, some children will develop COME without an antecedent history of AOM [7] The trigger that precipitates the onset of inflammation in these cases is unknown, but has been hypothesised to be low levels of bacteria entering the middle ear, sufficient to cause an inflammatory exudate, but not a purulent exudate [1].

Mahmood F Bhutta DPhil, FRCS (ORL-HNS), Clinical Lecturer and Specialist Registrar, UCL Ear Institute and University College London Hospitals, London, UK. Email: m.bhutta@doctors.org.uk (for correspondence)

Michael T Cheeseman DVM, PhD, FRCPath, Professor of Veterinary and Comparative Pathology, Neurobiology Division, Roslin Institute (University of Edinburgh), Edinburgh, UK

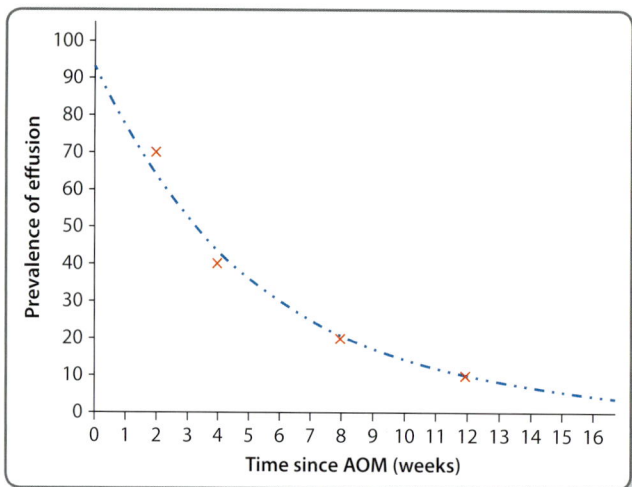

Figure 5.1 Prevalence of middle ear effusion following an episode of acute otitis media. Adapted from Bhutta [1], based on data from Teele et al. [6].

COME is unusual amongst chronic inflammatory diseases in that it is highly prevalent in childhood, and in that in most cases it resolves. Other chronic inflammatory disorders such as Crohn's disease, rheumatoid arthritis and multiple sclerosis usually develop in adulthood, and although they can show periods of remission, they rarely fully resolve. COME has been estimated to affect 1 in 18 of all children in the Western world during their second year of life [1], but longitudinal studies of affected children show that, in the majority, hearing normalises by late childhood or early adulthood (although otoscopic evidence of continuing middle ear disease may still be found) [8].

The ability of chronic OM to resolve suggests that there are changes in middle ear structure or function with age that enable that resolution, and that an understanding of these factors may allow targeted medical intervention. There is some evidence that persistent antigenic stimulation may play a role in non-resolution, in that culturable or non-culturable bacteria can be identified from most effusions of children with COME [1], and there is also some evidence of biofilm formation [9]. However, epidemiological studies exploiting twin and triplet siblings estimate that the heritability of time with middle ear effusion in early childhood is 71% [10]. This is strong evidence that there are factors intrinsic to the otitis prone child are the major determinants of chronicity of middle ear inflammation.

The traditional view of OM causation held that the susceptible child possessed an anatomical difference in the Eustachian tube. It has been suggested that because the tube is shorter, has a narrower calibre and is more horizontal in some children, this causes poor middle ear ventilation and OM susceptibility [11]. In this theory, an increasing length, calibre and angular orientation of the Eustachian tube with age facilitate disease resolution. Although this is an attractive hypothesis, an alternative interpretation of the evidence suggests that OME may cause Eustachian tube dysfunction via mucosa inflammation and lumen narrowing, rather than being the initial cause of OME. No studies show a consistent difference in the opening or closing pressure of the tube between otitis prone and normal children [12]. Abnormal opening or closing pressure can be demonstrated in some children when OME is present [13], but in children who have had a first episode of OME, Eustachian tube function does not correlate to disease recurrence [14], nor explain the success of surgical treatment [15,16]. However, preliminary results of balloon dilation of the Eustachian tube reported elsewhere in this book suggest that has therapeutic benefit, and so perhaps Eustachian tube narrowing may play some role in disease perpetuation.

It appears likely that polymorphisms in inflammatory response genes contribute to intrinsic susceptibility to chronic OM. As we understand more about chronic inflammatory diseases in a number of other organs, we have come to recognise that genetic susceptibility to these diseases often invokes shared molecular pathways [17]. It seems that similar key cytokines orchestrate the inflammatory response, and so perhaps a disruption of local regulators of these pathways can lead to organ-specific non-resolving inflammation [18], including in the middle ear. We have become particularly interested in the role of molecular pathways involved in the response to tissue hypoxia.

GAS EXCHANGE IN THE HEALTHY AND VENTILATED EAR

In the normal middle ear, ventilation occurs largely in the posterosuperior middle ear cleft [19] by transmucosal gaseous exchange between the middle ear space and venous blood [20–22]. The Eustachian tube plays little role in normal passive middle ear ventilation [23]. Consequently, the partial pressure of oxygen in the middle ear space mirrors that in venous blood, and is lower than that found in other healthy body organs at 39 mmHg (**Table 5.1**, **Figure 5.3**). Oxygen and carbon dioxide within cells (in middle ear mucosa, or leucocytes in effusion) are difficult to measure, but presumably will reflect loco-regional gaseous constitution. Hence, even the healthy middle ear is somewhat predisposed to hypoxia.

HYPOXIA PATHWAYS IN INFLAMMATION OF THE MIDDLE EAR

Ventilation of the middle ear is known to be an important factor in the resolution of chronic middle ear inflammation [25]. One possibility is that alleviation of hypoxia is an important mechanism underlying the therapeutic response and, by extension, hypoxia itself is a contributory factor in OM pathogenesis.

Hypoxia is a common feature of inflamed microenvironments [26,27]. Inflammation increases cellular energy demands, but at the same time tissue oedema and hyperplasia distances inflammatory cells from blood vessels and impairs oxygen delivery [28]. The master

Table 5.1 Partial pressures (mmHg) of gases in the healthy and surgically ventilated middle ear space*				
	Venous blood	Healthy middle ear	Air (37°C)	Middle ear after myringotomy
pO_2	38	39	150	138
pCO_2	44	48	0	15
H_2O	47	47	47	47
Inert gases	704	760	563	570
Total	704	760	760	760
*Data from Felding et al. [24].				

regulator of hypoxia response is the transcription factor hypoxia-inducible factor (HIF) [29]. Under conditions of normal oxygen, HIF protein level is degraded, but in hypoxic conditions the HIF protein becomes stabilised (**Figure 5.2**). HIF regulates a plethora of genes [30], and one of the key effectors is vascular endothelial growth factor (VEGF). HIF pathway activation affects cellular biosynthesis, extracellular matrix formation, glycolysis, energy production, cell survival, cell stress and promotes angiogenesis. These changes aid oxygen and nutrient delivery and improve cellular function under adverse conditions and so allow continued cellular function [31] and enable repair and restoration of tissue homeostasis [32]. However, persistent hypoxia signalling is maladaptive, and can contradictorily promote inflammation and tissue damage, and thus hinder rather than help resolution of inflammation [33].

HYPOXIA PATHWAYS IN ANIMAL MODELS OF OTITIS MEDIA AND CHILDREN WITH COME

The *Junbo* [34] and *Jeff* [35,36] mouse mutants carry point mutations in the *Evi1/Mecom* or *Fbxo11* genes respectively. In the *TGIF1* knockout mouse the gene is deleted [37]. These mouse mutants develop spontaneous chronic middle ear inflammation within a few weeks of birth. The mechanisms leading to chronic OM in the *Junbo, Jeff* and *TGIF1* mouse mutants are not fully understood but may be due in part to disrupted transforming growth factor beta signalling, which leads to a failure of the resolution phase of inflammation. Another mechanism in the *Junbo* mouse relates to the normal role of *Evi1/Mecom* as an inflammation-induced repressor of nuclear factor kappa beta (NFkB), the transcription factor that is a master regulator of inflammation. The *Junbo Evi1/Mecom* mutation confers a loss of function leading to de-repression of NFkB and predisposition to proinflammatory responses [38].

It is not entirely clear why spontaneous inflammatory disease is restricted to the middle ear in these mouse models, but it accords with the clinical observation that OM is very common in children in the absence of underlying immune compromise. This may relate to exposure to microbial challenge. The *Junbo* mouse does not have spontaneous lung pathology, but inflammatory responses of the lung are exaggerated when challenged with nontypeable *Haemophilus influenzae* [38]. The middle ear may be a sentinel site for inflammation because of its anatomy. Inflammatory cells accumulate within the

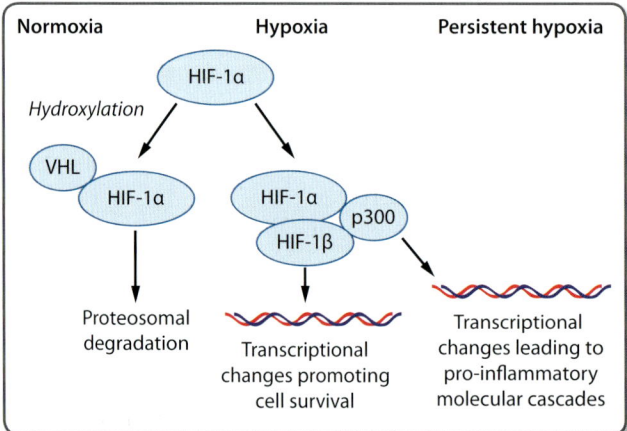

Figure 5.2 Hypoxia-inducible factor (HIF) signalling. Under conditions of normoxia, the HIF-1a subunit undergoes hydroxylation, which enables binding of von Hippel–Lindau protein and subsequent degradation. In hypoxia, HIF-1α is stabilised and binds HIF-1β and p300, and this unit then binds hypoxia responsive elements in transcriptional regulatory sites of a number of genes involved in cellular homeostasis and inflammation. Persistent signalling may become maladaptive.

bulla space, a large extra cellular compartment which is vulnerable to hypoxia and poor clearance of inflammatory cells.

The occurrence of hypoxia in the chronically inflamed middle ear can be demonstrated using in vivo labelling with pimonidazole (PIMO) which a small molecule marker of tissues with an oxygen tension below 10 mmHg ($\approx$1.5% O_2) [39]. The inflamed *Junbo* and *Jeff* bulla fluid inflammatory cells are labelled indicating it is physiologically hypoxic. In the *Junbo* mouse, (but not *Jeff*) middle ear mucosa is also labelled [40] (**Figure 5.4**).

In order to investigate gene expression in the inflamed middle ear, it is necessary to select a tissue for a baseline control. Healthy middle ears do not contain inflammatory cells in the bulla lumen and peripheral blood leucocytes (PBL) from the same mouse can serve as a control. PBL are not in an activated state or subject to the same prevailing hypoxic conditions in the inflamed ear. This PBL/bulla fluid leucocyte comparison was performed in *Junbo* and *Jeff* mouse mutants and showed relative upregulation of HIF-VEGF multiple signalling pathway genes (including HIF, VEGF and VEGF receptors). The levels of VEGF protein in the bulla fluids are increased >60-fold in the *Junbo*, *Jeff* and *TGIF* mice relative to serum VEGF protein [40].

HIF and VEGF pathways are also implicated in induced models of acute OM. VEGFA and VEGF receptor 1 (as well as FGF and FGFR1) are upregulated acutely in mice challenged with inoculation of nontypeable *Haemophilus influenzae* into the bulla [41] (the mouse equivalent of the mastoid). Middle ear HIF and VEGF are upregulated when OM is induced by Eustachian tube occlusion in the rat [42]. Osmotic minipump delivery of VEGF (and FGF) to the middle ear mucosa of the guinea pig leads to mucosal neovascularisation and middle ear effusion [41], and in a rabbit model of gastric content-induced middle ear inflammation, there is increased expression of VEGF [42].

Taken together, hypoxia-induced HIF-VEGF pathway activation appears to be a common feature in acute and chronic inflammatory disease of the middle ear in animal models. Two small-scale studies of adults and children with COME have reported VEGF presence in both effusions and mucosa [43,44], and presence of HIF has also been reported in COME [45]. We too have recently investigated hypoxia pathway activation in children undergoing grommet surgery for COME. Using the same experimental design as in the mouse studies (comparing PBL and glue ear inflammatory cells for gene expression, and serum and glue ear fluids for VEGF protein levels), we found comparable upregulation of multiple HIF-VEGF pathway genes as well as a consistent and marked elevation of VEGF protein (unpublished results).

MYRINGOTOMY TO ALLEVIATE HYPOXIA IN THE INFLAMED MIDDLE EAR

Ventilation of the healthy middle ear, through myringotomy with or without the insertion of a grommet (ventilation tube), exposes the middle ear to relative hyperoxia, such that in the ventilated middle ear oxygen pressures approach atmospheric levels (**Table 5.1**, **Figure 5.3**). Myringotomy in the inflamed middle ear may therefore raise middle ear oxygen tensions and have the effect of downregulating pathological hypoxia signalling.

The *Junbo* mouse model provides a means to test the hypothesis that the therapeutic effect of middle ear ventilation could, at least in part, be through the reversal of hypoxia. *Junbo* mice with bilateral OM underwent unilateral surgical myringotomy, and the middle ears were assessed by histology 5 days later comparing the operated and unoperated sides [46]. Myringotomy reduced middle ear inflammation, assessed by a smaller volume

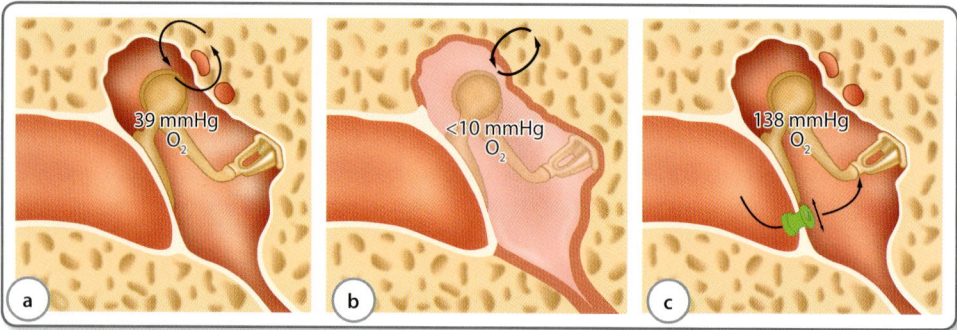

Figure 5.3 Hypothesised oxygenation in the healthy, chronically inflamed and ventilated middle ear. (a) In the healthy middle ear, oxygenation occurs largely as a result of transmucosal gas exchange with venous blood, leading to oxygen pressures of 39 mmHg. (b) In the chronically inflamed middle ear, there is tissue hypoxia because mucosal thickening impairs transmucosal gaseous exchange, and because inflammation consumes cellular oxygen. Data from mouse models suggests oxygen pressures may fall below 10 mmHg. (c) In the ventilated middle ear, there is relative hyperoxia as oxygen is introduced from the atmosphere, leading to oxygen pressures around 138 mmHg.

or resolved effusion, and by a statistically significant reduction in mucoperiosteal inflammatory thickening. *Junbo* mice that underwent unilateral myringotomy were labelled with PIMO, and in two of three mice PIMO labelling was absent in the operated ear, but still evident in the inflamed unoperated side (**Figure 5.4**).

Thus, reduction in chronic middle ear inflammation after myringotomy is associated with alleviation of tissue hypoxia. The goal of grommet insertion is the resolution of middle ear effusion, and a consequent improvement in hearing thresholds. In COME, the key constituent of the effusion are mucins, molecules formed of sugars and carbohydrates that give 'glue ear' its physical tenacity. Interestingly, the molecular regulation of mucin gene

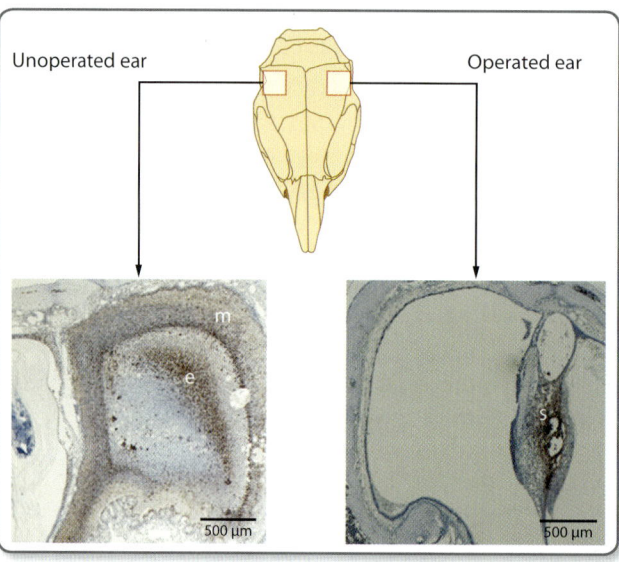

Figure 5.4 Effect of myringotomy on the Junbo mouse middle ear. Cross sections (x40) are stained brown with pimonidazole (PIMO), an adduct for tissues with pO2 <10 mmHg. In the normal unoperated middle ear, there is inflammation and thickening of the mucosa (m) with a leucocyte rich effusion (e). Both the mucosa and effusion stain with PIMO. In the operated ear, there is resolution of inflammation and effusion. PIMO labelling is evident only at the surgical site (s) of the healing tympanic membrane.

expression appears to be closely allied to hypoxia pathways. The *MUC5AC* gene encodes one of the major mucins found in COME [47], and studies in respiratory mucosa show one of its major promoters of transcription is the gene HIF [48]. If HIF expression is blocked, this can in turn abolish *MUC5AC* expression. Perhaps it is this molecular pathway that explains our clinical experience that middle ear ventilation causes a rapid and reliable resolution of middle ear effusion in COME.

MEDICAL TREATMENTS OF OTITIS MEDIA TARGETING HYPOXIA PATHWAYS

Prolonged HIF-VEGF signalling may be a major disease mechanism in OM. Angiogenesis in middle ear mucosa may predispose to vascular leak contributing to the accumulation of bulla fluids and inflammatory cells that in turn perpetuate the hypoxic conditions.

HIF-VEGF pathway members are major pharmacological targets in cancer therapies aimed at limiting tumour vascularisation. Small molecule inhibitors of VEGFR2 (the major receptor for VEGFA ligand) and HSP90 (a chaperone for HIF) act to limit tumour angiogenesis. Mouse models of OM are suitable for preclinical testing of compounds for efficacy in treating OM.

In a randomised controlled trial, *Junbo* mice were treated systemically with a VEGFR kinase inhibitor (either PTK-787, SU-11248 or BAY 43-9006) or a HSP-90 inhibitor (17-DMAG) once per day from day 28 to day 56. Treatment prevented progressive hearing loss in *Junbo* mice. PTK-787 reduces inflammatory thickening of the mucosal lining of the middle ear, and PTK-787, SU-11248 and 17-DMAG also reduce the occurrence of middle ear effusion [40].

Whilst this is encouraging, an important consideration in repurposing anticancer drugs for OM is that systemic treatment poses an unacceptable risk of toxicity in children. Medicating the middle ear directly is the most likely way forward, and an active area of research. For example, an eardrop formulation for transtympanic antibiotic delivery [49] has prospects for delivering other classes of compounds.

If realised, effective means to medicate the ear could revolutionise the treatment of middle ear disease by transferring treatment delivery to the primary health care system. Grommet insertion for COME remains the most common reason for childhood surgery in the Western world, and the consequences of chronic OM are still the major reason for tympanomastoidectomy. If in the future some of these operations could be prevented through medical therapies, perhaps targeting hypoxia pathways, the gain for our patients could be significant.

Key points for clinical practice

- Chronic otitis media has high heritability, implicating that host genetics plays a significant role in disease susceptibility.
- Ventilation of the healthy middle ear occurs largely through transmucosal gas exchange, and so oxygen pressures equilibrate with those in venous blood.
- Data from genetic mutant mouse models of otitis media demonstrate marked hypoxia and hypoxia gene upregulation in the chronically inflamed middle ear.
- Data from children with COME also show evidence of hypoxia gene upregulation.

- Surgical ventilation of a mouse model of chronic otitis media is associated with downregulation of inflammation and alleviation of tissue hypoxia.
- Experimental systemic therapy with antagonists of proteins involved in hypoxia response demonstrates resolution of inflammation and improved hearing in mouse models.
- Hypoxia pathways could be a target for future molecular therapy of chronic otitis media.

REFERENCES

1. Bhutta MF. Epidemiology and pathogenesis in otitis media: construction of a phenotype landscape. Audiol Neurotol 2014; 19:210-223.
2. Maw AR, Bawden R. Tympanic membrane atrophy, scarring, atelectasis and attic retraction in persistent, untreated otitis media with effusion and following ventilation tube insertion. Int J Pediatr Otorhinolaryngol 1994; 30:189–204.
3. Rudin R, Welin L, Svardsudd K, Tibblin G. Middle ear disease in samples from the general population. II. History of otitis and otorrhea in relation to tympanic membrane pathology. The study of men born in 1913 and 1923. Acta Otolaryngol 1985; 99:53–59.
4. Schilder AG, Zielhuis GA, Haggard MP, van den Broek P. Long-term effects of otitis media with effusion: otomicroscopic findings. Am J Otol 1995; 16:365–372.
5. Stangerup SE, Tos M, Arnesen R, Larsen P. A cohort study of point prevalence of eardrum pathology in children and teenagers from age 5 to age 16. Eur Arch Otorhinolaryngol 1994; 251:399-403.
6. Teele DW, Klein JO, Rosner BA. Epidemiology of otitis media in children. Ann Otol Rhinol Laryngol 1980; 89:5–6.
7. Alho OP, Oja H, Koivu M, Sorri M. Chronic otitis media with effusion in infancy. How frequent is it? How does it develop? Arch Otolaryngol Head Neck Surg 1995; 121:432–436.
8. Caye-Thomasen P, Stangerup SE, Jorgensen G, et al. Myringotomy versus ventilation tubes in secretory otitis media: eardrum pathology, hearing, and Eustachian tube function 25 years after treatment. Otol Neurotol 2008; 29:649–657.
9. Bakaletz LO. Bacterial biofilms in the upper airway - evidence for role in pathology and implications for treatment of otitis media. Paediatr Respir Rev 2012; 13:154–159.
10. Casselbrant ML, Mandel EM, Fall PA, et al. The heritability of otitis media: a twin and triplet study. JAMA 1999; 282:2125–2130.
11. Bluestone CD, Bluestone MB, Coulter J. The Eustachian tube: structure, function, role in otitis media. Hamilton: B C Decker; 2005.
12. de Ru JA, Grote JJ. Otitis media with effusion: disease or defense? A review of the literature. Int J Pediatr Otorhinolaryngol 2004; 68:331–339.
13. Takahashi H, Hayashi M, Sato H, Honjo I. Primary deficits in Eustachian tube function in patients with otitis media with effusion. Arch Otolaryngol Head Neck Surg 1989; 115:581–584.
14. Straetemans M, van Heerbeek N, Schilder AG, et al. Eustachian tube function before recurrence of otitis media with effusion. Arch Otolaryngol Head Neck Surg. 2005; 131:118–123.
15. Knight LC, Hilger A. The effects of grommet insertion on Eustachian tube function. Clin Otolaryngol Allied Sci 1993; 18:459–461.
16. van der Avoort SJ, van Heerbeek N, Zielhuis GA, Cremers CW. Sonotubometry in children with otitis media with effusion before and after insertion of ventilation tubes. Arch Otolaryngol Head Neck Surg 2009; 135:448–452.
17. Heap GA, van Heel DA. The genetics of chronic inflammatory diseases. Hum Mol Genet 2009; 18:R101–6.
18. Serhan CN, Brain SD, Buckley CD, et al. Resolution of inflammation: state of the art, definitions and terms. FASEB J 2007; 21:325–332.
19. Ars B, Wuyts F, Van de Heyning P, et al. Histomorphometric study of the normal middle ear mucosa. Preliminary results supporting the gas-exchange function in the posterosuperior part of the middle ear cleft. Acta Otolaryngol 1997; 117:704–707.
20. Doyle WJ, Seroky JT. Middle ear gas exchange in rhesus monkeys. Ann Otol Rhinol Laryngol 1994; 103:636–645.
21. Hamada Y, Utahashi H, Aoki K. Physiological gas exchange in the middle ear cavity. Int J Pediatr Otorhinolaryngol 2002; 64:41–49.

22. Sade J, Ar A. Middle ear and auditory tube: middle ear clearance, gas exchange, and pressure regulation. Otolaryngol Head Neck Surg 1997; 116:499–524.
23. Sade J, Cinamon U, Ar A, Seifert A. Gas flow into and within the middle ear. Otol Neurotol 2004; 25:649–652.
24. Felding JU, Rasmussen JB, Lildholdt T. Gas composition of the normal and the ventilated middle ear cavity. Scand J Clin Lab Invest Suppl 1987; 186:31–41.
25. Takahashi H. The middle ear: the role of ventilation in disease and surgery. Tokyo: Springer-Verlag; 2001.
26. Dehne N, Brune B. HIF-1 in the inflammatory microenvironment. Exp Cell Res 2009; 315:1791–1797.
27. Frede S, Berchner-Pfannschmidt U, Fandrey J. Regulation of hypoxia-inducible factors during inflammation. Methods Enzymol. 2007; 435:405–419.
28. Nizet V, Johnson RS. Interdependence of hypoxic and innate immune responses. Nat Rev Immunol 2009; 9:609–617.
29. Coleman ML, Ratcliffe PJ. Oxygen sensing and hypoxia-induced responses. Essays Biochem 2007; 43:1–15.
30. Benita Y, Kikuchi H, Smith AD, et al. An integrative genomics approach identifies Hypoxia Inducible Factor-1 (HIF-1)-target genes that form the core response to hypoxia. Nucleic Acids Res. 2009; 37:4587–4602.
31. Walmsley SR, Cadwallader KA, Chilvers ER. The role of HIF-1alpha in myeloid cell inflammation. Trends Immunol 2005; 26:434–439.
32. Siddiq A, Aminova LR, Ratan RR. Hypoxia inducible factor prolyl 4-hydroxylase enzymes: center stage in the battle against hypoxia, metabolic compromise and oxidative stress. Neurochem Res 2007; 32:931–946.
33. Ikeda E. Cellular response to tissue hypoxia and its involvement in disease progression. Pathol Int 2005; 55:603–610.
34. Parkinson N, Hardisty-Hughes RE, Tateossian H, et al. Mutation at the Evi1 locus in Junbo mice causes susceptibility to otitis media. PLoS Genetics 2006; 2:e149.
35. Hardisty RE, Erven A, Logan K, et al. The deaf mouse mutant Jeff (Jf) is a single gene model of otitis media. J Assoc Res Otolaryngol. 2003; 4:130–138.
36. Hardisty-Hughes RE, Tateossian H, Morse SA, et al. A mutation in the F-box gene, Fbxo11, causes otitis media in the Jeff mouse. Hum Mol Genet 2006; 15:3273–3279.
37. Tateossian H, Morse S, Parker A, et al. Otitis media in the Tgif knockout mouse implicates TGFβ signalling in chronic middle ear inflammatory disease. Hum Mol Genet 2013;22:2553-65.
38. Xu X, Woo CH, Steere RR, et al. EVI1 Acts as an Inducible Negative-Feedback Regulator of NF-kappaB by Inhibiting p65 Acetylation. J Immunol 2012; 188:6371–6380.
39. Kizaka-Kondoh S, Konse-Nagasawa H. Significance of nitroimidazole compounds and hypoxia-inducible factor-1 for imaging tumor hypoxia. Cancer Sci 2009; 100:1366–1373.
40. Cheeseman MT, Tyrer HE, Williams D, et al. HIF-VEGF pathways are critical for chronic otitis media in Junbo and Jeff mouse mutants. PLoS Genet 2011; 7:e1002336.
41. Husseman J, Palacios SD, Rivkin AZ, Oehl H, Ryan AF. The role of vascular endothelial growth factors and fibroblast growth factors in angiogenesis during otitis media. Audiol Neurootol 2012; 17:148–154.
42. Huang Q, Zhang Z, Zheng Y, et al. Hypoxia-inducible factor and vascular endothelial growth factor pathway for the study of hypoxia in a new model of otitis media with effusion. Audiol Neurootol 2012; 17:349–356.
43. Sekiyama K, Ohori J, Matsune S, Kurono Y. The role of vascular endothelial growth factor in pediatric otitis media with effusion. Auris Nasus Larynx 2011; 38:319–324.
44. Jung HH, Kim MW, Lee JH, et al. Expression of vascular endothelial growth factor in otitis media. Acta Otolaryngol 1999; 119:801–808.
45. Zhou H, Chen ZB, Tian HQ, et al. Effects of hypoxia-inducible factor 1alpha on bone conduction impairment in otitis media with effusion. Acta Otolaryngol 2012; 132:938–943.
46. Bhutta MF, Cheeseman MT, Brown SDM. Myringotomy in the Junbo mouse model of chronic otitis media alleviates cellular hypoxia and inflammation. Laryngoscope 2014; 124:E377-383.
47. Kerschner JE, Tripathi S, Khampang P, Papsin BC. MUC5AC expression in human middle ear epithelium of patients with otitis media. Arch Otolaryngol Head Neck Surg 2010; 136:819–824.
48. Young HW, Williams OW, Chandra D, et al. Central role of Muc5ac expression in mucous metaplasia and its regulation by conserved 5′elements. Am J Respir Cell Mol Biol 2007; 37:273–290.
49. Khoo X, Simons EJ, Chiang HH, et al. Formulations for trans-tympanic antibiotic delivery. Biomaterials 2013; 34:1281–1288.

Chapter 6

Balloon dilation Eustachian tuboplasty

Holger Sudhoff, Jörg Ebmeyer, Stefanie Schröder, Martin Lehmann

INTRODUCTION

The Eustachian tube (ET) is part of a system including the nose, palate, rhinopharynx and middle ear space. This comprises the middle ear cleft, which includes the bony ET, tympanic cavity and the mastoid air cell system (**Figure 6.1**). The tympanic cavity and mastoid cells are interconnected and allow for gas exchange and pressure regulation. The ET is a complex organ consisting of a dynamic canal with its mucosa, cartilage, surrounding soft tissue, peritubal muscles (i.e. tensor and levator veli palatini, salpingopharyngeus and tensor tympani) and superior bony support and the sphenoid sulcus.

Clinical experience as well as numerous patient studies and animal models show that the ET plays an important role in middle ear pathology [1–3]. Our knowledge of the mechanical properties of the ET has improved significantly in recent years, but uncertainties persist due to its complex anatomy, the variety of functions of the organ and the impact of intrinsic and external factors on its function [4,5]. Intermittent transitory tubal dilation is probably the major mechanism for equilibration of middle ear cleft pressure with the ambient atmosphere [6]. Barometric and chemical receptors within the middle ear cleft are assumed to provide autonomic nervous system feedbacks that impact the frequency of involuntary tubal opening [7,8]. However, transmucosal gas exchange is also recognised as important for middle ear ventilation, and the gaseous constituents of the normal middle ear reflect that of venous blood [9]. Our understanding of the anatomy and physiology of the ET continues to evolve. Recently, McDonald et al. showed that the ET may have a sequential peristaltic-like mechanism [10].

Eustachian tube dysfunction (ETD) can lead to clinical symptoms such as aural fullness, impaired pressure equilibration, altered middle ear aeration, hearing loss and autophony [11]. Because the most common cause of obstructive dysfunction is mucosal inflammation

Holger Sudhoff MD, PhD, FRCS, FRCPath, Professor and Chairman, Department of Otolaryngology, Head and Neck Surgery, Bielefeld Academic Teaching Hospital, Münster University, Bielefeld, Germany
Email: holger.sudhoff@rub.de (for correspondence)

Jörg Ebmeyer MD, Department of Otolaryngology, Head and Neck Surgery, Bielefeld Academic Teaching Hospital, Münster University, Bielefeld, Germany

Stefanie Schröder MD, Department of Otolaryngology, Head and Neck Surgery, Bielefeld Academic Teaching Hospital, Münster University, Bielefeld, Germany

Martin Lehmann Department of Otolaryngology, Head and Neck Surgery, Bielefeld Academic Teaching Hospital, Münster University, Bielefeld, Germany

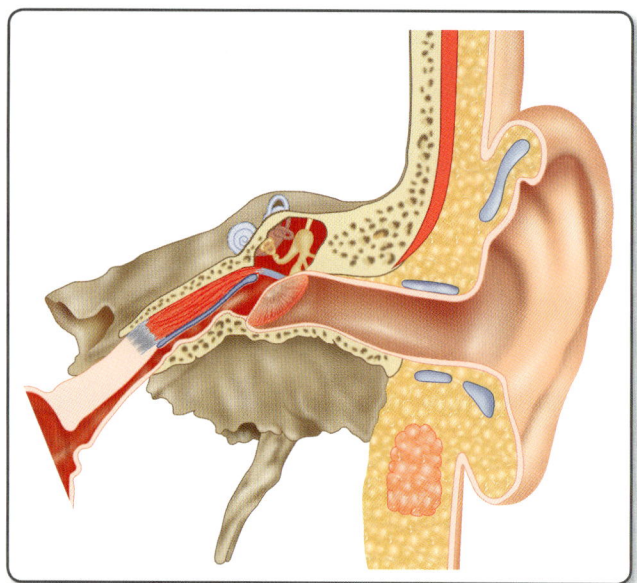

Figure 6.1 Temporal bone drawing comprising the middle ear cleft, the bony and cartilaginous Eustachian tube, tympanic cavity and the mastoid air cell system.

within the cartilaginous ET, patients should be questioned about inflammatory processes that could contribute, including allergic rhinitis, chronic rhinosinusitis, laryngopharyngeal reflux and smoke exposure [12,13]. Paediatric ETD may be caused by adenoid tissue and mucosa swelling due to acute or chronic upper respiratory tract infections. Cleft palate, granulomatous diseases, cystic fibrosis, Samter's triad and primary ciliary dyskinesia are potential contributing factors. ET function may be a contributing factor to vertigo [12]. It is important to distinguish ETD from other causes of aural fullness such as patulous ET, temporomandibular joint disorders, superior semicircular canal dehiscence syndrome, Meniere's disease and increased intracranial pressure.

The incidence of ETD in adults is estimated at 1% of the general population [13]. Studies accessing paediatric and adult patient cohorts demonstrate that ETD is detectable in up to two-thirds of patients undergoing middle ear surgery [14,15]. Regain of ET function is believed to be important for the success of middle ear surgery [16–20].

HISTORY OF TREATMENT OF THE EUSTACHIAN TUBE

The ET has been investigated ever since the Greek physician and philosopher Alkmaion of Kroton mentioned its existence in 500 BC. Detailed knowledge about its anatomy and physiology was obtained by the work of Bartholomeus Eustachius, Antonio Maria Valsalva, Joseph Toynbee and several other otologists [21]. One of the first suggestions to treat ETD was forwarded by the French postal employee E.G. Guyot in 1724. He used a knee-shaped bent tin tube, positioned it via the mouth into the torus tubarius, and flushed the ET several times. Antoine Saissy (1752–1822) evolved Guyot's concept into bougienage of the ET using a gut string [21]. In 1969, W.F. House introduced an invasive approach to Eustachian tuboplasty via a middle fossa approach. None of these procedures were associated with long-term success, and so were abandoned [22].

Recently interest in treatment of the ET has regained in popularity. Technological advancements have enabled novel surgical interventions including balloon dilation tuboplasty, laser tuboplasty and microdebrider tuboplasty. Long-term results with these experimental procedures are not yet established, but early results show promise [23–29].

DEVELOPMENT OF BALLOON DILATION EUSTACHIAN TUBOPLASTY

Our group has developed Balloon dilation Eustachian Tuboplasty (BET) as a novel treatment option directed at the proposed cause of chronic otitis media. Our concept was inspired by dilatation of the arterial vessel lumen in percutaneous transluminal coronary angioplasty and balloon sinuplasty. The aim of this minimally invasive intervention is a dilatation of the cartilaginous part of the ET. It was clinically applied for the first time in 2008 and is currently adopted by >80 otological departments across Europe [24].

Our group first undertook feasibility and safety studies of BET in human cadavers. Five human cadaveric ETs were treated with a 600 µm diameter balloon catheter inflated with a pressure of 10 bar for 2 minutes (**Figure 6.2**). The balloon could always be placed correctly into the ET. High-resolution computed tomography (CT) scans with three-dimensional reconstruction were used to verify correct placement of the balloon catheter, and fine-cut temporal bone histology was performed. We found no obvious complications, and specifically no injury to the internal carotid artery (ICA). Microscopic tears were visible in the cartilaginous part of the ET [23].

We improved our BET method with a softer and more flexible balloon and a special insertion tool. In 2008, we undertook our first clinical study of BET in eight adults with chronic ETD who had previously undergone tympanoplasty. The procedures were without complication and enabled us to standardise our technique [23,24].

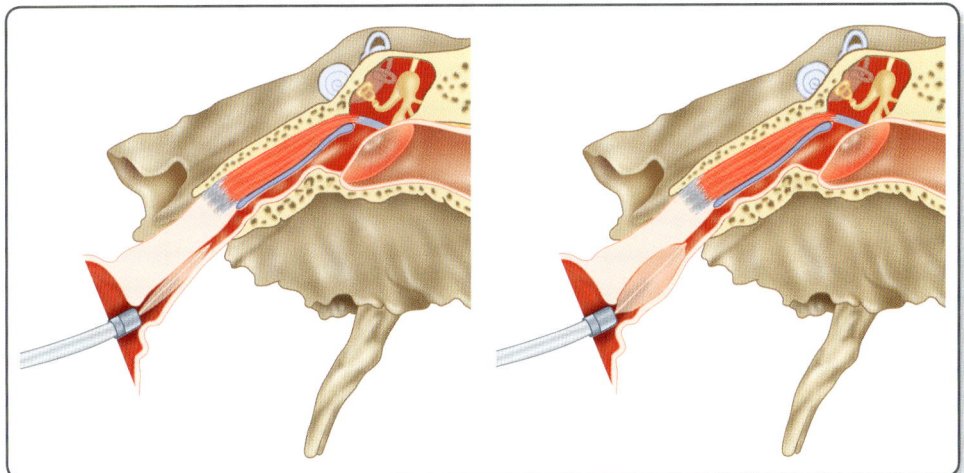

Figure 6.2 The balloon catheter inserted into the cartilaginous Eustachian tube (left) and inflated with a pressure of 10 bar for two minutes (right).

TECHNIQUE FOR BET

We recommend BET is performed with the patient under general anaesthesia [24]. There are three different approaches to intubate the ET:

1. The catheter insertion tool with an integrated microendoscope is positioned transnasally into the nasopharyngeal ET ostium and the catheter advanced into the cartilaginous part of the ET, and is designed to prevent too deep insertion (**Figure 6.3**)

2. An insertion device can also be used, and catheterisation of the ET visualised with either a 45° or 70° Hopkins endoscope in the contralateral nostril or a 30° Hopkins endoscope in the ipsilateral nostril (**Figure 6.4**)

3. In cases with significant nasal septal deviation, a transoral 70° endoscope with velotraction can be used to visualise the nasopharynx. This can also be achieved with a flexible endoscope or an angled mirror, as used in adenoidectomy (**Figure 6.5**). The tool offers three differently angled extensions for differing anatomy: 30°, 45° and 70° (**Figure 6.6**)

Once the catheter is inserted into the ostium of the ET, the balloon is inflated with saline to 10 bar for 2 minutes to dilate the cartilaginous part of the ET. The balloon has defined dimensions of 2.0 cm in length and 3.28 mm in diameter at 10 bars. Careful observation of the extraction of the catheter from the ET after dilation gives feedback as to whether the catheter was really inside the tube, and not kinked in the mucosal folds of the nasopharynx, e.g. the fossa of Rosenmuller.

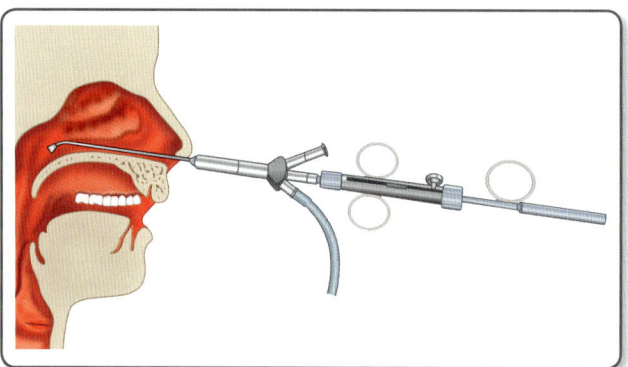

Figure 6.3 The catheter insertion tool with an integrated microendoscope is introduced into the nasopharyngeal Eustachian tube (ET) ostium and the catheter advanced into the cartilaginous part of the ET.

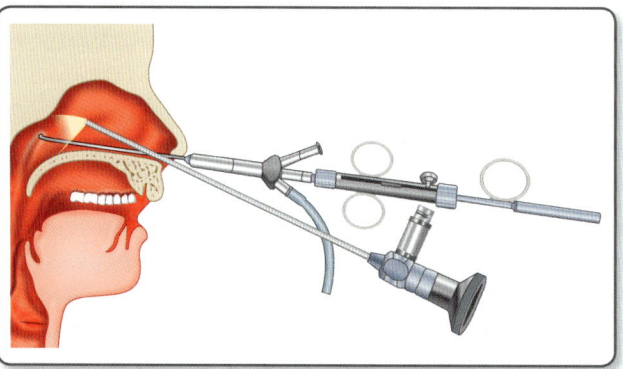

Figure 6.4 An insertion device and catheterisation of the Eustachian tube visualised with a 45° or 70° Hopkins endoscope in the contralateral nostril or a 30° Hopkins endoscope in the ipsilateral nostril.

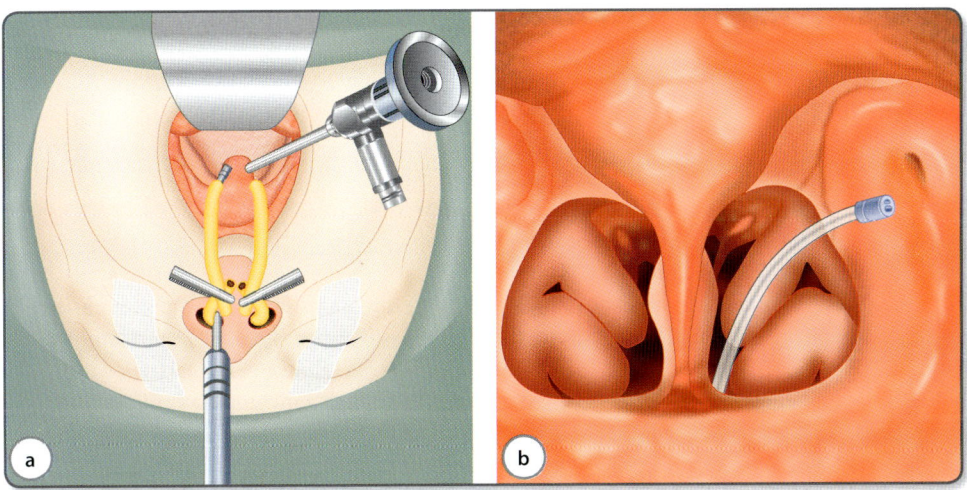

Figure 6.5 (a) Significant nasal septal deviation may require a transorally inserted 70° endoscope with velotraction. (b) This can also be achieved with a flexible endoscope or an angled mirror, as used in adenoidectomy.

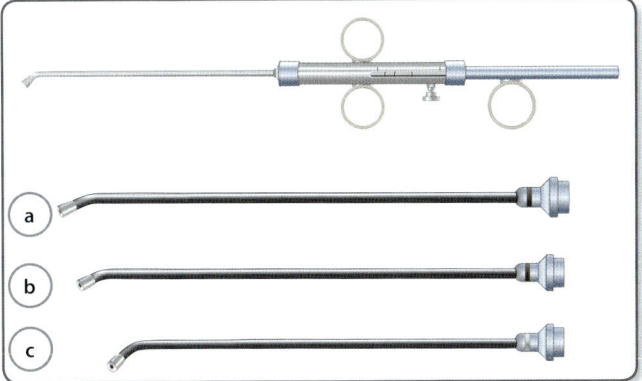

Figure 6.6 Novel insertion tool with three angled extensions: (a) 30°, (b) 45° and (c) 70°, colour coded according to Hopkins endoscopes.

ASSESSMENT OF EUSTACHIAN TUBE FUNCTION

In the assessment of patients with ETD, symptoms of ear pressure or problems with pressure equalisation can be combined with clinical tests such as otoscopy, otoendoscopy, the Politzer's test or the Valsalva's and Toynbee's manoeuvres. More formal tests of ET function are usually used only for research. More than 40 methods to assess ET function have been described [30], but none have been proven to measure all aspects of ET physiology or pathology.

Manometric tests of ET function include tympanometry, reflex decay tympanometry, the nine-step inflation deflation test, the modified inflation deflation test, the forced response test and tubomanometry (TMM) [30–33]. The pressure chamber is an ideal device to evaluate ET function, whether the tympanic membrane is intact or perforated. Sonotubometry utilises sound delivered via a probe in the nose, whilst recording changes in sound amplitude in the external ear canal resulting from tube opening. Other approaches to assess ET function include phototubometry, scintigraphy, ultrasound, application of dye or taste-bearing substances, electromyography, flow measurements and (opto)tensometry [30]. None of these methods is yet clinically proven [31].

We evaluate ET function through criteria based on the ETDQ-7 questionnaire and TMM. The ETDQ-7 questionnaire (**Table 6.1**), developed by McCoul et al. in 2012, asks patients to score the severity of a number of pressure-related symptoms in their ears, with a suggested cut-off point of 14.5 for diagnosing ETD [34].

TMM, described by Estève in 2001 [35,36], involves the controlled delivery of pressures of 30, 40 and 50 mbar to the nasopharynx through a nasal applicator. Swallowing triggers opening of the cartilaginous part of the ET, and a pressure receptor probe in the external auditory canal registers pressure changes transmitted though movement of the tympanic membrane, or through a perforation in the tympanic membrane. If the ET opens during swallowing, the pressure applied to the nasopharynx is transmitted to the middle ear. Pressure curves of the nasopharynx and the ear canal are displayed on a monitor and allow calculation of a number of parameters (**Figure 6.7**). The opening latency index (R value) is the latency between pressure application in the nasopharynx and recording of a pressure change in the ear canal [35]. Immediate opening ($R<1$) indicates good ET function, and late opening ($R>1$) indicates restricted ET function. No opening (R negative or not measurable) indicates complete obstruction of the ET. In contrast to older TMM methods, this technique is feasible whether a tympanic perforation is present or not and delivers specific information about the dynamics of the ET.

Our overall rating of ET function is with a Eustachian tube score, incorporating clinical symptoms and TMM results, i.e. subjective and objective data (**Table 6.2**). The clinical symptoms 'clicking sound when swallowing' and 'positive Valsalva's manoeuvre' are rated 0 for 'never', 1 for 'sometimes' and 2 for 'always'. TMM results, specifically R values at 30, 40 and 50 mbar, are also incorporated into the ET score. Immediate opening of the ET ($R \leq 1$) is weighted with 2 points, delayed opening ($R>1$) with 1 point and no opening (negative or not measurable R) with 0 points. The summation of these five tests yields an ET score between 0 (worst value) and 10 (best value). The ET score gives a single quantitative

Table 6.1 The ETDQ-7 questionnaire

Over the past 1 month, how much has each of the following been a problem for you?	No problem		Moderate problem			Severe problem	
1. Pressure in the ears?	1	2	3	4	5	6	7
2. Pain in the ears?	1	2	3	4	5	6	7
3. A feeling that your ears are clogged or 'under water'?	1	2	3	4	5	6	7
4. Ear symptoms when you have a cold or sinusitis?	1	2	3	4	5	6	7
5. Crackling or popping sounds in the ears?	1	2	3	4	5	6	7
6. Ringing in the ears?	1	2	3	4	5	6	7
7. A feeling that your hearing is muffled?	1	2	3	4	5	6	7

It is a tool for the evaluation of chronic obstructive Eustachian tube dysfunction [34].

able to perform the Valsalva's manoeuvre. At 2 months 67% of patients have symptomatic improvement, and 71% at 6 months. There was a 2% revision rate.

SAFETY OF BET

In our hands, we have found BET to usually be a straightforward procedure and have not observed any serious complications with its use [40]. In >700 BET procedures, three patients developed preauricular emphysema, presumably as a result of an ET mucosal tear. In all three cases, the emphysema resorbed under antibiotic cover and the ET healed without evidence of permanent damage, and indeed with improvement in ET function. The only other adverse effects observed thus far are minor bleeding, and a temporary increase in pre-existing tinnitus for 2 weeks after the procedure. Others have also reported haemotympanum and C6–C7 radiculopathy [41]. Patulous ET has never been observed in our series of BET [39,40].

We have debated the necessity of preoperative high-resolution CT scanning of the temporal bone in predicting complications of BET [42]. CT will provide information on the relationship between the ET and the bony canal of the ICA, but represents a significant dose of radiation. We initially feared that dilation, although performed within the cartilaginous part of the ET, might affect the bony part of the ET, possibly leading to plaque mobilisation within the ICA, or fractures of the thin bony canal with penetration of bony fragments into the ICA, causing cerebrovascular accident or fatal bleeding. There could also be direct trauma in the case of ICA dehiscence in the temporal bone.

Moreano et al. examined 1000 temporal bones and reported carotid canal dehiscence in 77 cases and microdehiscences in a further 74 cases. Thus, in their series 15.5% of carotid canals had no or only thin bony coverage [43]. Tisch et al. also evaluated CT scans of 1000 patients but reported no dehiscence of the carotid canal, in their series, with a mean thickness of the carotid canal of 1.02 mm [38]. Our own study of 284 CT scans of the temporal bone before unilateral or bilateral BET found radiological carotid canal dehiscence in 18 cases (6.3%), but in no case did injury to the carotid artery ensue. In three patients in this series (4 ETs), balloon dilation could not be performed due to difficulties advancing the balloon catheter, but preoperative CT scan was not helpful in predicting such failure [42]. We now do not recommend preoperative CT scanning.

FUTURE WORK

ETD is often been regarded as a 'black box' in which the function of the system remains unclear. We now understand that there are a variety of underlying reasons leading to ETD. We believe identification and treatment of ETD is crucial to achieving clinical improvement in chronic ear disease.

BET seems to be a promising option in the treatment of ETD. Our initial data demonstrate that BET is a safe method, and that the majority of patients show improvement in objective and subjective measures of ETD. Our results are mirrored by smaller case series from other authors. Data on clinical outcomes requires longer follow-up, but in some of our patients we have observed resolution of middle ear effusion, reversal of tympanic retraction and healing of tympanic perforations. It would be useful to compare such outcomes in randomised trials.

Additional studies may help us to identify subgroups of patients that are most likely to benefit from this procedure, and so enable the development of relevant inclusion and exclusion criteria. The role of this procedure in treating middle ear effusion in nasopharyngeal carcinoma or in patients with cleft palate is not clear. Studies in children have not yet been performed. Regardless of these shortcomings, our current data suggest that BET could play a significant future role in the treatment of chronic ear disease.

Key points for clinical practice

- Balloon dilation of the cartilaginous, ET is a feasible alternative to tympanostomy tube placement in patients with chronic obstructive ETD.
- The ETDQ-7 questionnaire helps as an instrument for the evaluation of ET function. TMM is a clinical exploration method that measures pressure transmission from the nasopharynx to the middle ear.
- The ET score combines clinical symptoms with the outcomes of TMM to assess ET function.
- Preoperative high-resolution CTs of the temporal bones are not routinely recommended.
- Patients with problems of pressure equilibration or chronic otitis media are potential candidates for BET.
- Results demonstrate that BET is a safe and effective treatment for improving ET function and middle ear ventilation in adults.
- Further studies are required in order to establish this treatment in terms of clinical outcomes, and to define its role in the management of children.

REFERENCES

1. Leuwer R, Koch U. Anatomy and physiology of the auditory tube. Therapeutic possibilities in chronic disorders of tubal function. HNO 1999; 47:514–523.
2. Bluestone CD. Introduction. In: Bluestone MB (ed.), Eustachian tube: structure, function, role in otitis media. Hamilton, Ontario: BC Decker; 2005:1–9.
3. Sudhoff H. Eustachian tube dysfunction. Uni-Med Verlag Bremen, London, Boston: UNI-MED; 2013.
4. Seibert JW, Danner CJ. Eustachian tube function and the middle ear. Otolaryngol Clin North Am 2006; 39:1221–1235.
5. Pau HW. Eustachian tube and middle ear mechanics. Acta Otolaryngol 2011; 131:1279–1285.
6. Sadé J, Luntz M, Levy D. Middle ear gas composition and middle ear aeration. Ann Otol Rhinol Laryngol 1995; 104:369–373.
7. Eden A, Gannon P. Neural control of middle ear aeration. Arch Otolaryngol Head Neck Surg 1987; 113:133–137.
8. Rockley T, Hawke W. The middle ear as a baroreceptor. Acta Otolaryngol 1992; 112:816–823.
9. Doyle WJ, Yuksel S, Banks J, Alper CM. Directional asymmetry in the measured nitrous oxide time constant for middle ear transmucosal gas exchange. Ann Otol Rhinol Laryngol 2007; 116:69–75.
10. McDonald MH, Hoffman MR, Gentry LR, Jiang JJ. New insights into mechanism of Eustachian tube ventilation based on cine computed tomography images. Eur Arch Otorhinolaryngol 2012; 269:1901–1907.
11. Bluestone CD, Klein JO. Otitis media, atelectasis, and Eustachian tube dysfunction. In: Bluestone CD, Stool SE, Kenna MA (eds), Pediatric otolaryngology, 3rd edn. Philadelphia: WB Saunders; 1996.
12. Takahashi H, Honjo I, Fujita A. Endoscopic findings at the pharyngeal orifice of the Eustachian tube in otitis media with effusion. Eur Arch Otorhinolaryngol 1996; 253:42–44.
13. Poe DS, Gopen Q. Eustachian tube dysfunction. In: Snow JB, Wackym PA, Ballenger JJ (eds), Ballenger's otorhinolaryngology: head and neck surgery. Lewiston, New York: BC Decker; 2009:201–208.
14. Browning GG, Gatehouse S. The prevalence of middle ear disease in the adult British population. Clin Otolaryngol Allied Sci 1992; 17:317–321.

15. Gudziol V, Mann WJ. Chronic Eustachian tube dysfunction and its sequelae in adult patients with cleft lip and palate. HNO 2006; 54:684–688.
16. Goldman JL, Martinez SA, Ganzel TM. Eustachian tube dysfunction and its sequelae in patients with cleft palate. South Med J 1993; 86:1236–1237.
17. Mewes T, Mann W. Function of the Eustachian tube in epitympanic retraction pockets. HNO 1998; 46:914–918.
18. Choi SH, Han JH, Chung JW. Pre-operative evaluation of Eustachian tube function using a modified pressure equilibration test is predictive of good postoperative hearing and middle ear aeration in type 1 tympanoplasty patients. Clin Exp Otorhinolaryngol 2009; 2:61–65.
19. Podoshin L, Fradis M, Malatskey S, Ben-David J. Tympanoplasty in adults: a five-year survey. Ear Nose Throat J 1996; 75:149–152, 155–166.
20. Dorrie A, Dommerich S, Pau HW. Early postoperative middle-ear ventilation -- risk for the transplant or guarantee for aeration of the tympanic cavity? Laryngorhinootologie 2003; 82:102–104.
21. Mudry A. In reference to evolution of Eustachian tube surgery. Laryngoscope 2012; 122:939–940.
22. House WF, Glasscock ME 3rd, Miles J. Eustachian tuboplasty. Laryngoscope 1969; 79:1765–1782.
23. Ockermann T, Reineke U, Upile T, Ebmeyer J, Sudhoff H. Balloon dilatation Eustachian tuboplasty (BET): a feasibility study. Otology Neurotol 2010; 31:1100–1103.
24. Ockermann T, Reineke U, Upile T, Ebmeyer J, Sudhoff H. A clinical study: balloon dilatation Eustachian tuboplasty (BET). Laryngoscope 2010; 120:1411–1416.
25. Caffier PP, Sedlmaier B, Haupt H, et al. Impact of laser Eustachian tuboplasty on middle ear ventilation, hearing, and tinnitus in chronic tube dysfunction. Ear Hear 2011; 32:132-139.
26. Poe DS, Grimmer JF, Metson R. Laser Eustachian tuboplasty: two-year results. Laryngoscope 2007; 117:231–237.
27. Kujawski OB, Poe DS. Laser Eustachian tuboplasty. Otol Neurotol 2004;25:1–8.
28. Poe DS, Silvola J, Pyykkö I. Balloon dilation of the cartilaginous Eustachian tube. Otolaryngol Head Neck Surg 2011; 144:563–569.
29. Metson R, Pletcher SD, Poe DS. Microdebrider Eustachian tuboplasty: a preliminary report. Otolaryngol Head Neck Surg 2007; 136:422–427.
30. Di Martino E, Thaden R, Krombach GA, Westhofen M. Function tests for the Eustachian tube. Current knowledge. HNO 2004; 52:1029–1040.
31. Todd NW. There are no accurate tests for Eustachian tube function. Arch Otolaryngol Head Neck Surg 2000; 126:1041–1042.
32. Sudhoff H, Ockermann T, Mikolajczyk R. Clinical and experimental considerations for evaluation of Eustachian tube physiology. HNO 2009; 57:428–435.
33. Poe DS, Pyykkö I. Measurements of Eustachian tube dilation by video endoscopy. Otol Neurotol 2011; 32:794–798.
34. McCoul ED, Anand VK, Christos PJ. Validating the clinical assessment of Eustachian tube dysfunction: the Eustachian Tube Dysfunction Questionnaire (ETDQ-7). Laryngoscope 2012; 122:1137–1141.
35. Esteve D, Dubreuil C, Della Vedova C, Normand B, Martin C. Evaluation par tubomanometrie de la fonction douverture tubaire et de la réponse tympanique chez le sujet normal et chez le sujet porteur dune otide séro-muqueuse chronique. J Fr ORL 2001; 50:223–231.
36. Ars B, Dirckx, JJ. Tubomanometry. Den Haag: Kugler; 2003.
37. Tisch M, Maier S, Hecht P, Maier H. Bilateral Eustachian tube dilation in infants: an alternative treatment for persistent middle ear functional dysfunction. HNO 2013; 61:492–493.
38. Tisch M, Störrle P, Danz B, Maier H. Role of imaging before Eustachian tube dilation using the Bielefeld balloon catheter. HNO 2013; 61:488–491.
39. Sudhoff H, Schröder S, Reineke U, et al. Therapy of chronic Eustachian tube dysfunction. Evolution of applied therapies. HNO 2013; 61:477–482.
40. Schröder S, Reineke U, Lehmann M, Ebmeyer J, Sudhoff H. Chronic obstructive Eustachian tube dysfunction in adults. Long-term results of balloon Eustachian tuboplasty. HNO 2013; 61:142–151.
41. Miller BJ, Elhassan HA. Balloon dilatation of the Eustachian tube: an evidence based review of case series for those considering its use. Clin Otolaryngol 2013. doi: 10.1111/coa.12195.
42. Abdel-Aziz T, Schröder S, Lehmann M, et al. Computed tomography prior to balloon Eustachian tuboplasty – a true necessity? Otology Neurotol 2014;35: 635-638.
43. Moreano EH, Paparella MM, Zelterman D, Goycoolea MV. Prevalence of microfissures in the human temporal bone: a report of 1000 temporal bones. Laryngoscope 1994; 104:741–746.

Chapter 7

Superior canal dehiscence syndrome

Rupan Banga, Richard Irving

INTRODUCTION

The concept of superior canal dehiscence syndrome (SCDS) was first introduced in 1998 by Lloyd Minor et al. [1]. They described eight patients with auditory as well as vestibular symptoms that were evoked by sound or pressure applied to the ear. Previously these patients were either thought to have a psychosomatic illness or may even have undergone a variety of treatments for other otological conditions [2]. The symptoms are generated by a mobile third window effect of the dehiscent superior semicircular canal (SSC)[2].

AETIOLOGY

SCDS is caused by a dehiscence of the bone covering the SSC in the middle cranial fossa (MCF). Rarely the posterior semicircular canal may be involved [3].

Carey et al. [4] microscopically examined 1000 temporal bones in nearly 600 adults and found that the incidence of dehiscence of the bone overlying the superior canal was 0.5% of the temporal bones (or 0.7% of individuals). Interestingly, an additional 1.4% of specimens (0.7% of individuals) had bone that was <0.1 mm in thickness, which might appear dehiscent even on high-resolution imaging. The most common sites for dehiscence were in the MCF floor, or in a deep groove for the superior petrosal sinus.

It is unclear whether this anatomic abnormality is developmental or acquired. SCDS has been described in children, supporting a developmental aetiology [5–7]. It has been postulated that as the membranous and osseous labyrinths are near adult size early in fetal development, there is a disproportion in the size of the labyrinth compared with the rest of the skull base causing a protrusion of the SSC into the MCF. This protrusion may cause adhesion of the membranous labyrinth to the MCF dura prior to complete ossification occurring [8].

However, most patients with SCDS present later in life and often after an episode of trauma, barotrauma or straining. Perhaps the MCF dura acts as a plug and patients only present after trauma which causes the MCF adhesion to lift off the SSC [8]. However, a

Rupan Banga MBChB, FRCS (ORL-HNS), PhD, Consultant Otologist, University Hospital Birmingham, Birmingham, UK. Email: rupan@doctors.org.uk (for correspondence)

Richard Irving FRCS(ORL-HNS), Consultant Otologist, University Hospital Birmingham, Birmingham, UK

study carried out in Boston demonstrated that prevalence of SSC dehiscence on imaging positively correlated with increasing age [9]. This would favour an acquired aetiology, with the mechanism of thinning presumably related to dural pulsations over a long period of time. It is important to note that not all patients with a dehiscence noted on imaging are symptomatic.

PATHOGENESIS

The auditory symptoms may be explained by the effects on the inner ear of a third mobile window. Air conduction thresholds are increased because some of the sound energy from the vibration of the stapes footplate is diverted along a path of least resistance, away from the cochlea, up through the superior canal and out through the dehiscence. The mobile third window also affects the compressional mechanism of bone conduction, whereby the mobile third window increases the impedance between the scala tympani and scala vestibuli. This causes the basilar membrane to vibrate more easily and hence increases the response of the cochlea to bone-conducted sound [10]. The raised thresholds for air-conducted sound and reduced thresholds for bone-conducted sound lead to a pseudoconductive hearing loss [2,11].

Under normal circumstances, there is minimal fluid displacement in the vestibular apparatus in response to noise. In patients with SCDS, the mobile third window created by the dehiscence allows greater volume displacement, which can lead to inadvertent stimulation of vestibular sensors within the membranous labyrinth in response to noise. Similar responsiveness to pressure changes applied to the external ear can also occur. These give rise to characteristic sound and pressure evoked eye movements, because of stimulation of the vestibulo-ocular reflex [1,12].

SYMPTOMS

A characteristic early feature of SCDS is autophony, with patients commonly reporting that they can hear their own footsteps, joint and even eye movements. This is likely to be due to a hyperacusis of bone-conducted sound. The condition may be misdiagnosed as Eustachian tube dysfunction or patulous Eustachian tube. In addition, patients may have been previously diagnosed with otosclerosis if a conductive deficit is present [13,14]. Other auditory symptoms that are frequently reported include aural fullness and pulsatile tinnitus. Vestibular symptoms may arise as a result of sound or pressure-induced vertigo and occasionally oscillopsia or positional vertigo [15].

SIGNS

The ears are usually otoscopically normal, but it may be possible to elicit nystagmus with tragal pressure (Henebert's sign) or by exposing the ear to loud sound (Tullio phenomenon). Positive pressure in the external auditory canal and Valsalva's manoeuvre against closed nostrils displaces the cupula of the affected SSC in an excitatory direction causing vertical–torsional nystagmus, with a slow phase component directed superiorly and a torsional component rotating away from the stimulated ear. Conversely, Valsalva against a closed glottis deflects the SSC in its inhibitory direction. Patients with a bilateral symptomatic dehiscence may demonstrate a vertical downbeat nystagmus with no torsional component on Valsalva, this being cancelled out due to the simultaneous stimulation of both sides [16]. Tuning fork tests may suggest a conductive hearing loss in the affected ear, the Weber test typically lateralising to the affected ear. In bilateral cases this may not occur.

INVESTIGATIONS

Pure tone audiometry

Pure tone audiometry typically gives a picture of pseudoconductive hearing loss, with negative bone conduction thresholds in the lower frequencies, occasionally down to –15 dB (see **Figure 7.1**). There is evidence that the size of the air-bone gap correlates to the size of the dehiscence [17]. The stapedial reflexes elicited by air-conducted sound remain normal, differentiating SCDS from an ossicular chain fixation [18].

Vestibular evoked myogenic potential

The vestibular evoked myogenic potential (VEMP) is a short latency muscle relaxation potential that is created when the vestibular system is stimulated with loud sound (**Figure 7.2**). It represents the response of the otolith organs. The myogenic potential is most commonly recorded from the sternocleidomastoid muscle [cervical (cVEMP)], but can also be recorded from other muscle groups including the inferior ocular muscles [ocular (oVEMP)] and the masseter.

Clinically, the cVEMP is most frequently utilised with air-conducted sound as this is thought to specifically evoke an ipsilateral saccular response. The pathway is a manifestation of the vestibulocollic reflex: a stimulus to the saccule is transmitted to the vestibular nucleus in the brainstem via the inferior vestibular nerve. The efferent

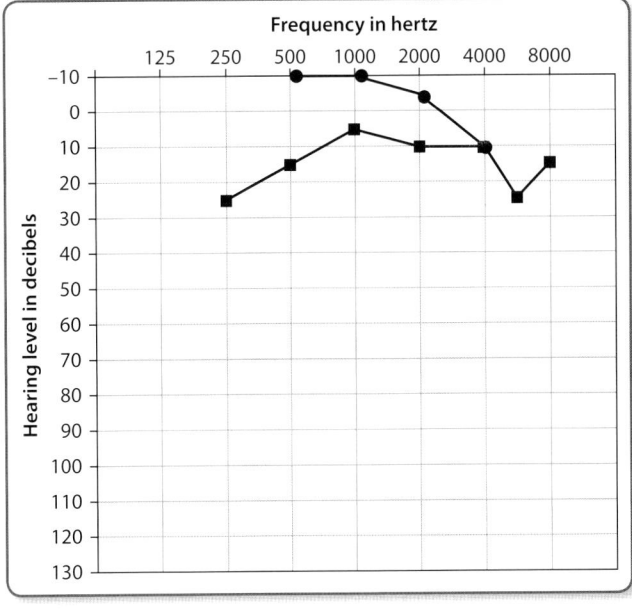

Figure 7.1 Pure tone audiogram demonstrating pseudoconductive hearing loss in a patient with right superior canal dehiscence (squares indicate left unmasked air conduction and circles indicate left masked bone conduction).

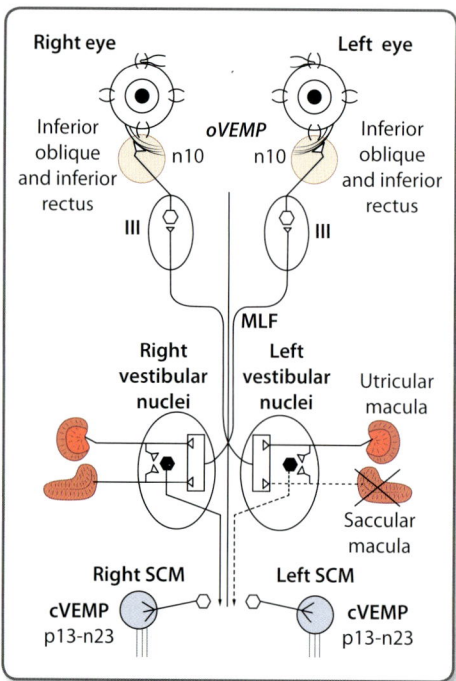

Figure 7.2 Schematic diagram of some of the known vestibulo-ocular and vestibulocollic projections which underlie the ocular and cervical vestibular evoked myogenic potential (oVEMP and cVEMP) responses to bone-conducted vibration delivered to the midline forehead at the hairline. From Manzari et al. [41].

pathway is via the medial vestibulospinal tract to the neck musculature [19]. cVEMP responses are the short latency relaxation potentials measured from tonically contracting sternocleidomastoid muscles that relax in response to ipsilateral presentation of loud click noises [20]. Normative data on cVEMP responses show changes with ageing, with a decrease in cVEMP amplitude and increase in cVEMP threshold with increasing age [21].

Patients with SCDS will usually demonstrate low threshold cVEMP responses (<70 dB threshold) with a much larger amplitude on the affected side if the pathology is unilateral [22]. VEMP testing has been found to normalise after surgical plugging of the dehiscence [23].

The oVEMP measures the extraocular electromyographic activity associated with the vestibulo-ocular reflex. It is thought to be a crossed pathway involving the vestibular nerve and nucleus, transmitted via the medial longitudinal fasciculus, the oculomotor nuclei and nerves, to the extraocular muscles [19].

Imaging

Temporal bone computed tomographic (CT) scans with 0.5 mm collimation and reconstruction in the plane of the SSC and orthogonal to the SSC are the gold standard for identification of dehiscence [24]. There is some concern that current CT imaging overestimates the incidence and size of SCD due to partial volume averaging. There are a number of studies reporting incidence of SCD on CT of 3–8% compared with 0.5–1.4% in cadaveric studies [4,25–29].

Multiplanar reconstructions of high-resolution CT data are the most sensitive test for the diagnosis of SCD and are more accurate than three-dimensional surface reconstructions of the temporal bone [30]. The positive predictive value of CT scanning can be increased from 50% to 93% by using fine slice protocols and reformatting images in the plane of and at 90°

to the SSC [24]. However, in larger series it seems that even when using submillimetre slices with oblique reformats, the actual positive predictive value is much lower, between 57% and 67% [25] (see **Figure 7.3**).

DIAGNOSIS AND MANAGEMENT

The diagnosis of SCDS relies upon the correlation of characteristic symptoms and signs with physiological findings and radiological imaging. As temporal bone CT imaging can overestimate the incidence of SCDS, it is vital that the radiological findings are considered in conjunction with the history and clinical findings.

In patients with minimal symptoms, thorough explanation of the condition with avoidance of provoking stimuli is usually sufficient to limit disability. Some patients will present with symptoms that are having a profound effect on their quality of life. If there is a good clinical suspicion of SCDS, supported by audiological testing and imaging, then surgical treatment to plug or resurface the dehiscence may be considered.

Minor et al. originally described a classical MCF craniotomy and extradural approach to resurface or plug the SSC from above [2,31,32]. Transmastoid middle fossa craniotomy repair has also been described. After a cortical mastoidectomy, the dura surrounding the area of dehiscence is exposed and elevated, and tragal perichondrium is used to repair or plug the defect [33]. Resurfacing or plugging can also be achieved using fascia, bone chips or hydroxyapatite cement. A meta-analysis from 2009 suggests that canal plugging is more effective than canal resurfacing [34].

More recently a transmastoid canal plugging approach has been reported [34–39]. A standard cortical mastoidectomy is performed and the SSC identified. The anterior and posterior limbs are blue lined (bone removed to expose the endosteum), the semicircular canal endostium is depressed using a blunt needle and the dehiscence is isolated from the rest of the labyrinth by plugging each limb with fascia and small bone fragments. In some cases, the MCF floor may be too low to access the SSC via a transmastoid route, in which case either the classical or transmastoid middle fossa craniotomy approaches can be used.

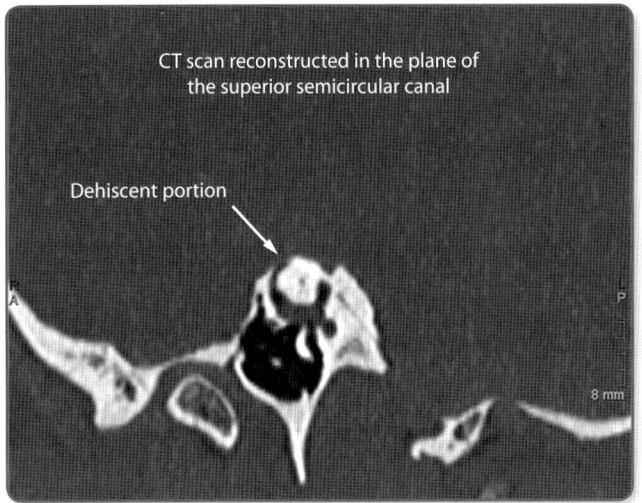

Figure 7.3 A computed tomography scan of the right temporal bone reconstructed in the plane of the semicircular canal. The dehiscence is arrowed.

We favour a transmastoid canal plugging approach where possible as it is faster and avoids the risks and complications associated with a craniotomy and temporal lobe retraction.

RESULTS

Most patients experience a degree of imbalance in the immediate postoperative period and should be counselled to this effect. This is usually best addressed with vestibular therapy; however, a small proportion may have more protracted imbalance. In addition, patients may experience an initial transient postoperative hearing loss, which is typically mixed in nature. The postoperative hearing preservation varies in the literature. Minor's team report that in those patients with a preoperative low-frequency air-bone gap, the gap typically decreases after surgical plugging via the MCF approach, and that 25% of patients have a persistent high-frequency sensorineural hearing loss postoperatively with no change in speech discrimination [40]. This is thought to be a result of loss of perilymph during the surgical procedure. Zhao et al. report no significant postoperative hearing loss following a series of 11 transmastoid canal plugging procedures [37]. The full auditory benefits may not be apparent for up to 6 weeks after surgery; however, often patients report an immediate improvement in autophony.

CONCLUSION

As with all disorders of balance, the diagnosis of SCDS relies heavily on the clinical history. A patient who can hear their eyeballs moving, whose Weber test lateralises to the symptomatic ear, along with the other features previously described, should raise the index of suspicion for SCDS. Imaging can be difficult to interpret and we feel strongly that high-resolution CT scanning should not be used as a diagnostic test, but used in conjunction with other findings. VEMP testing can also be misleading, particularly in bilateral cases.

If the surgeon is confident of the diagnosis and the patient describes the symptoms as having a significant impact on their quality of life, then surgery is a very reasonable option in an appropriately informed patient. Complete resolution of all symptoms might be unrealistic, but significant or full resolution of symptoms can be achieved with surgery in the majority of appropriately selected cases in our experience.

Key points for clinical practice

- The diagnosis of SCDS relies on a good clinical history supported by clinical examination findings.
- High resolution CT scanning and and VEMP testing are useful adjuncts but should not be used solely as diagnostic tests.
- Many patients can be treated conservatively but if a surgical approach is required, the transmastoid canal plugging technique avoids the morbidity associated with the MCF approach.

REFERENCES

1.   Minor LB, Solomon D, Zinreich JS, Zee DS. Sound- and/or pressure-induced vertigo due to bone dehiscence of the superior semicircular canal. Arch Otolaryngol Head Neck Surg 1998; 124:249–258.
2.   Minor LB, Carey JP, Cremer PD, et al. Dehiscence of bone overlying the superior canal as a cause of apparent conductive hearing loss. Otol Neurotol 2003; 24:270–278.

3. Whyte J, Cisneros AI, Martinez C, et al. Congenital dehiscence in the posterior semicircular canal. Otol Neurotol 2013; 34:1134–1137.
4. Carey JP, Minor LB, Nager GT. Dehiscence or thinning of bone overlying the superior semicircular canal in a temporal bone survey. Arch Otolaryngol Head Neck Surg 2000; 126:137–147.
5. Chen EY, Paladin A, Phillips G, et al. Semicircular canal dehiscence in the pediatric population. Int J Pediatr Otorhinolaryngol 2009; 73:321–327.
6. Zhou G, Ohlms L, Liberman J, Amin M. Superior semicircular canal dehiscence in a young child: implication of developmental defect. Int J Pediatr Otorhinolaryngol 2007; 71:1925–1928.
7. Lee GS, Zhou G, Poe D, et al. Clinical experience in diagnosis and management of superior semicircular canal dehiscence in children. Laryngoscope 2011; 121:2256–2261.
8. Takahashi N, Tsunoda A, Shirakura S, Kitamura K. Anatomical feature of the middle cranial fossa in fetal periods: possible etiology of superior canal dehiscence syndrome. Acta Otolaryngol 2012; 132:385–390.
9. Nadgir RN, Ozonoff A, Devaiah AK, Halderman AA, Sakai O. Superior semicircular canal dehiscence: congenital or acquired condition? AJNR Am J Neuroradiol 2011; 32:947–949.
10. Merchant SN, Rosowski JJ, McKenna MJ. Superior semicircular canal dehiscence mimicking otosclerotic hearing loss. Adv Otorhinolaryngol 2007; 65:137–145.
11. Limb CJ, Carey JP, Srireddy S, Minor LB. Auditory function in patients with surgically treated superior semicircular canal dehiscence. Otol Neurotol 2006; 27:969–980.
12. Cremer PD, Minor LB, Carey JP, Della Santina CC. Eye movements in patients with superior canal dehiscence syndrome align with the abnormal canal. Neurology 2000; 55:1833–1841.
13. Lehmann M, Ebmeyer J, Upile T, Sudhoff HH. Superior canal dehiscence in a patient with three failed stapedectomy operations for otosclerosis: a case report. J Med Case Rep 2011; 5:47.
14. Li PM, Bergeron C, Monfared A, Agrawal S, Blevins NH. Superior semicircular canal dehiscence diagnosed after failed stapedotomy for conductive hearing loss. Am J Otolaryngol 2011; 32:441–444.
15. Brantberg K, Bergenius J, Mendel L, et al. Symptoms, findings and treatment in patients with dehiscence of the superior semicircular canal. Acta Otolaryngol 2001; 121:68–75.
16. Chien WW, Carey JP, Minor LB. Canal dehiscence. Curr Opin Neurol 2011; 24:25–31.
17. Yuen HW, Boeddinghaus R, Eikelboom RH, Atlas MD. 15th Yahya Cohen Memorial Lecture - the relationship between the air-bone gap and the size of superior semicircular canal dehiscence. Ann Acad Med Singapore 2011; 40:59–64.
18. Carey JP, Migliaccio AA, Minor LB. Semicircular canal function before and after surgery for superior canal dehiscence. Otol Neurotol 2007; 28:356–364.
19. Rosengren SM, Welgampola MS, Colebatch JG. Vestibular evoked myogenic potentials: past, present and future. Clin Neurophysiol 2010; 121:636–651.
20. Streubel SO, Cremer PD, Carey JP, Weg N, Minor LB. Vestibular-evoked myogenic potentials in the diagnosis of superior canal dehiscence syndrome. Acta Otolaryngol Suppl 2001; 545:41–49.
21. Janky KL, Shepard N. Vestibular evoked myogenic potential (VEMP) testing: normative threshold response curves and effects of age. J Am Acad Audiol 2009; 20:514–522.
22. Brantberg K, Bergenius J, Tribukait A. Vestibular-evoked myogenic potentials in patients with dehiscence of the superior semicircular canal. Acta Otolaryngol 1999; 119:633–640.
23. Welgampola MS, Myrie OA, Minor LB, Carey JP. Vestibular-evoked myogenic potential thresholds normalize on plugging superior canal dehiscence. Neurology 2008; 70:464–472.
24. Belden CJ, Weg N, Minor LB, Zinreich SJ. CT evaluation of bone dehiscence of the superior semicircular canal as a cause of sound- and/or pressure-induced vertigo. Radiology 2003; 226:337–343.
25. Cloutier JF, Belair M, Saliba I. Superior semicircular canal dehiscence: positive predictive value of high-resolution CT scanning. Eur Arch Otorhinolaryngol 2008; 265:1455–1460.
26. Masaki Y. The prevalence of superior canal dehiscence syndrome as assessed by temporal bone computed tomography imaging. Acta Otolaryngol 2011; 131:258–262.
27. Sequeira SM, Whiting BR, Shimony JS, Vo KD, Hullar TE. Accuracy of computed tomography detection of superior canal dehiscence. Otol Neurotol 2011; 32:1500–1505.
28. Stimmer H, Hamann KF, Zeiter S, Naumann A, Rummeny EJ. Semicircular canal dehiscence in HR multislice computed tomography: distribution, frequency, and clinical relevance. Eur Arch Otorhinolaryngol 2012; 269:475–480.
29. Tavassolie TS, Penninger RT, Zuniga MG, Minor LB, Carey JP. Multislice computed tomography in the diagnosis of superior canal dehiscence: how much error, and how to minimize it? Otol Neurotol 2012; 33:215–222.
30. Crane BT, Minor LB, Carey JP. Three-dimensional computed tomography of superior canal dehiscence syndrome. Otol Neurotol. 2008; 29:699–705.

31. Minor LB. Superior canal dehiscence syndrome. Am J Otol. 2000; 21:9–19.
32. Minor LB. Clinical manifestations of superior semicircular canal dehiscence. Laryngoscope 2005; 115:1717–1727.
33. Teixido M, Seymour PE, Kung B, Sabra O. Transmastoid middle fossa craniotomy repair of superior semicircular canal dehiscence using a soft tissue graft. Otol Neurotol 2011; 32:877–881.
34. Vlastarakos PV, Proikas K, Tavoulari E, et al. Efficacy assessment and complications of surgical management for superior semicircular canal dehiscence: a meta-analysis of published interventional studies. Eur Arch Otorhinolaryngol 2009; 266:177–186.
35. Agrawal SK, Parnes LS. Transmastoid superior semicircular canal occlusion. Otol Neurotol 2008; 29:363–367.
36. Deschenes GR, Hsu DP, Megerian CA. Outpatient repair of superior semicircular canal dehiscence via the transmastoid approach. Laryngoscope 2009; 119:1765–1769.
37. Zhao YC ST, van Dinther J, Vanspauwen R, Husseman J, Briggs RJ. Transmastoid repair of superior semicircular canal dehiscence. J Neurol Surg Part B 2012; 73:225–229.
38. Wijaya C, Dias A, Conlon BJ. Superior semicircular canal occlusion-Transmastoid approach. Int J Surg Case Rep 2012; 3:42–44.
39. Shaia WT, Diaz RC. Evolution in surgical management of superior canal dehiscence syndrome. Curr Opin Otolaryngol Head Neck Surg 2013; 21:497–502.
40. Ward BK, Agrawal Y, Nguyen E, et al. Hearing outcomes after surgical plugging of the superior semicircular canal by a middle cranial fossa approach. Otol Neurotol 2012; 33:1386–1391.
41. Manzari L, Burgess AM, Curthoys IS. Ocular and cervical vestibular evoked myogenic potentials in response to bone-conducted vibration in patients with probable inferior vestibular neuritis. J Laryngol Otol 2012; 126:683–691.

Chapter 8

Regeneration of hair cells in the inner ear: possibilities and challenges

Jonathan E Gale, Stephanie Juniat, Ruth R Taylor, Andrew Forge

INTRODUCTION

Loss of the sensory 'hair' cells from the organ of Corti – the auditory epithelium of the mammalian cochlea – is a major cause of hearing loss. In addition, the loss of hair cells in the vestibular sensory epithelia – the utricular and saccular maculae and the cristae of the semicircular canals – is a significant factor in balance dysfunction. In the mammalian cochlea, hair cell loss, which in many cases is progressive, is followed by a delayed but progressive loss of the afferent neurons that synapse with the hair cells. It is worth noting that in some cases, e.g. auditory neuropathy, simply put, the loss of innervation may be the primary effect. The latter is important to note since cochlear implants rely upon the continued presence of auditory nerves; consequently such neuronal loss can compromise the efficacy of the prosthesis.

In all non-mammalian vertebrates studied to date – i.e. birds, reptiles, amphibians and fish – when hair cells, either auditory or vestibular, die they are spontaneously replaced by new ones (see [1] for review), the replacement cells become innervated and there is essentially complete recovery of function. In mammals, although an ability to regenerate or replace hair cells in the vestibular sensory epithelia has been demonstrated [2,3], the regenerative capacity is severely limited. In the case of the mature mammalian cochlea, there is no hair cell regeneration. Consequently in mammals the functional deficits resulting from death of hair cells – hearing loss or balance disequilibrium – are permanent. In recent years, a greater understanding of not only the molecular pathways involved in otic development, e.g. genes specifying inner ear tissues and determining hair cell production, but also the mechanisms that underlie hair cell regeneration in mature sensory epithelia from non-mammalian vertebrates have established a basis for regenerative strategies to

Jonathan E Gale PhD, Reader in Auditory Cell Biology, UCL Ear Institute, 332 Gray's Inn Road, London, UK. Email: jonathan.gale@ucl.ac.uk (for correspondence)

Stephanie Juniat graduate student, UCL Ear Institute, 332 Gray's Inn Road, London, UK.

Ruth R Taylor PhD Research Fellow, UCL Ear Institute, 332 Gray's Inn Road, London, UK.

Andrew Forge PhD, Professor of Auditory Cell Biology, UCL Ear Institute, 332 Gray's Inn Road, London, UK.

replace lost hair cells and/or neurons in the mammal. There are broadly two suggested approaches: to induce hair cell regeneration 'endogenously' in a manner similar to that which occurs in nonmammalian vertebrates; or to use 'exogenous' cells derived from stem cells that will differentiate in situ in the inner ear as hair cells or neurons.

THE CELLULAR ORGANISATION OF THE SENSORY EPITHELIA OF THE INNER EAR

Sensory epithelia of the inner ear in all vertebrates have mechanosensitive hair cells that are surrounded by and separated from their neighbours by nonsensory supporting cells (**Figure 8.1a-b**). In the mammalian cochlea, the organ of Corti, whilst conforming to this same general principle, shows particular cell-architectural specialisations related to the differentiated status of the supporting cells *(***Figure 8.1c-d***)*. In the organ of Corti, hair cells are established in rows, with a single row of inner hair cells (IHC) and three, sometimes four, more lateral but parallel rows of outer hair cells (OHC) (**Figure 8.1c-d**). IHC are the primary receptor cells that send auditory signals to the brain and they are innervated by

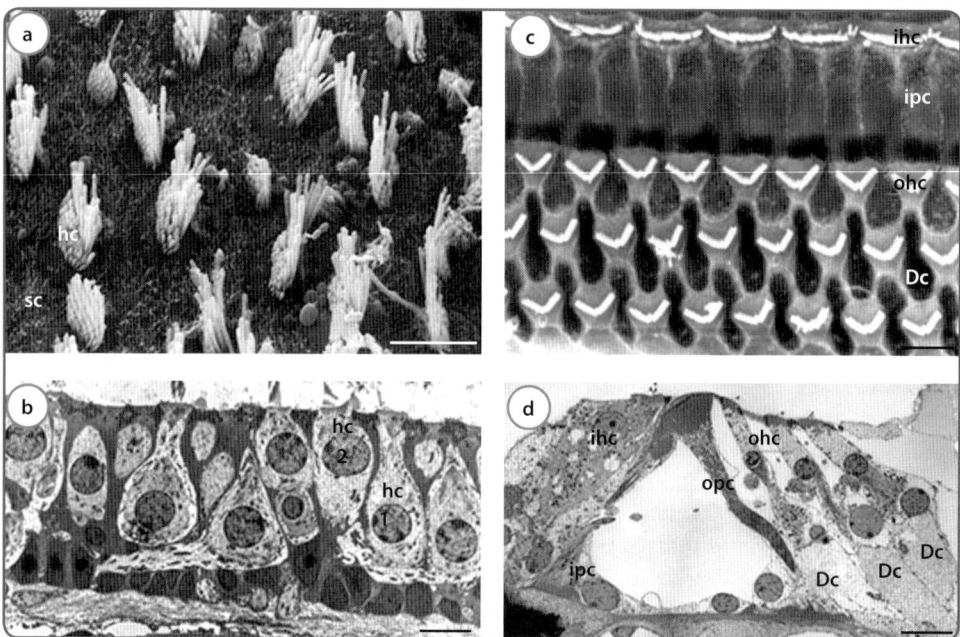

Figure 8.1 Sensory epithelia of the mammalian inner ear. (a) Scanning electron microscopy of the luminal surface of the utricular macula shows the hair bundles on each hair cell (hc). Each hc is surrounded and separated by supporting cells (sc), the surfaces of which are covered in microvilli. (b) Cross-section of the utricular macula reveals two hc types: the flask-shaped type 1 (hc1) and cylindrical type 2 (hc2). The bodies of the supporting cells (sc) from a layer at the basal aspect of the epithelium and their projections to the luminal surface separate hc from each other. (c) Scanning electron microscopy of the luminal surface of the organ of Corti shows the single row of inner hair cells (ihc) and three rows of outer hair cells (ohc). The heads of the inner pillar cells (ipc) separate the row of ihc from the first row of ohc. The heads of Deiters' cells (Dc) intervene between ohc. (d) Cross-section of the organ of Corti shows ipc and opc that delineate the tunnel of Corti separating the ihc from the ohc and Dc in the region of the ohc. Supporting cells of the organ of Corti, like the equivalent cells in the vestibular system, have their cell bodies located below the hc and send projections to the luminal surface between the hc. Scale bars: 10 µm.

the majority of the cochlear afferent nerves, each IHC synapsing with several (ca. 10–15) individual afferent fibres. The OHC, on the other hand, are the cellular basis of cochlear amplification. Their motile activity, driven in response to mechanical stimulation, feeds back to enhance the sound-induced vibrations of the cochlear basilar membrane leading to amplification of the mechanical input to the IHC. The supporting cells of the organ of Corti – including the Deiters' cells that surround the OHC, and the pillar cells that separate the region of OHC from that of the IHC – are structurally specialised to provide the mechanically rigid environment necessary for the amplification process [4-6]. Those supporting cell specialisations are particular to the organ of Corti, and are not apparent either in the inner ears of other vertebrates or in the mammalian vestibular sensory epithelia. In the organ of Corti, and in fact all other hair cell epithelia, supporting cells also play a primary role in maintaining the physiological environment (homeostasis), particularly of the fluid environment that is necessary for effective hair cell function and survival. Despite there being no direct evidence for a role in potassium recycling, there is a significant weight of indirect data and models that suggest that supporting cells ensure that the concentration of potassium ions around the hair cell bodies is kept to physiological levels under normal conditions. High potassium ion concentration in the spaces around hair cells not only compromises the ionic gradients essential for signal transduction by hair cells but also can be toxic. Mutations in the genes that encode many of the proteins involved in potassium homeostasis that are expressed by supporting cells can result in death of hair cells, particularly OHC [7-9]. Having functional supporting cells is thus a significant consideration for strategies aimed at regenerating hair cells; if the physiological environment in which hair cells are regenerated is abnormal or cannot be maintained, those replacement hair cells may not survive.

RELEVANT CONSIDERATIONS OF INNER EAR DEVELOPMENT

The development and maturation of the inner ear requires the coordinated expression of specific genes and genetic networks (**Figure 8.2**). Formation of the otic vesicle, the primordial structure that gives rise to the inner ear, is defined by a specific set of genes, and once this has been generated, the expression of other genes further defines the location of sensory and nonsensory domains. Within the domains that will become the auditory and vestibular sensory epithelia, cells are specified as sensorineural progenitors. They undergo cell division, and some of the cells are specified as neural precursors. Further cell division of the neural precursors is inhibited by specific cell cycle regulatory proteins and the precursors exit the cell cycle, migrate out of the otic vesicle epithelium and differentiate as afferent neurons. These delaminated cells group together forming nascent structures that will become the cochlear spiral ganglion and the vestibular ganglion. Axons from these cells extend toward the developing brain, and others toward the developing sensory epithelium. Other daughter cells from division of the sensorineural progenitors undergo one additional and final cell division to create the sensory precursors in which mitosis is terminally halted through expression of the cell cycle regulatory protein p27kip1 [10,11]. The daughter cells of these terminal mitotic events differentiate without further cell division into either hair cells or supporting cells. Cells which go on to become hair cells express a transcription factor Atoh1 (atonal homologue type1, previously known as Math1) which acts to regulate the expression of the genes that determine the hair cell fate. In mice in which the Atoh1 gene has been ablated, hair cells do not form in either the organ of Corti or vestibular sensory epithelia [12.13]. Consequently, Atoh1 expression is considered necessary for a cell in the inner ear to differentiate as a hair cell. Atoh1 has also been shown to be sufficient to determine hair cell fate at least when expressed in inner ear cells [13,14]. Sensorineural progenitor cells that begin to differentiate in this way inhibit their immediate neighbours from following the same fate; they express proteins of the 'Delta' family, ligands that bind to their corresponding 'Notch' receptors in the membrane of adjacent cells. The binding of Delta to Notch activates a pathway that suppresses differentiation as a hair cell so the inhibited cell becomes a supporting cell [15,16]. Note that in this developmental sequence, hair and supporting cells derive from a common precursor cell and afferent neurons derive from the same cell lineage as hair and supporting cells [17,18].

The expression of p27kip1, a cell-cycle inhibitor, follows the exit from the cell cycle that is observed in mammalian sensory epithelia [11]. As hair cells begin to differentiate, expression of p27kip1 is downregulated and a different inhibitor of cell cycle progression, phosphorylated retinoblastoma protein (pRb), is expressed [19,20]. Supporting cells continue to be held in mitotic arrest by the expression of p27kip1. Also, as hair cells differentiate, they will begin to produce certain 'neurotrophins', chemicals that attract neurites from the auditory nerve toward them so the sensory cells become innervated (see [21] for review). The continued production of neurotrophins by hair cells (and also by some supporting cells) in the mature organ of Corti is important for the survival of neurons throughout the life of an animal. This is likely to be the primary reason why loss of hair cells is followed by loss of neurons.

During the earliest stages of development of the organ of Corti, hair cell specification is also regulated by other factors. The width of the sensory domain, as defined by the number of cells expressing p27Kip1 in sensory precursors, is wider than the stripe of cells that will constitute the mature organ of Corti [11,22]. In the cochlea, the number of hair cells generated in the initial stages of organ of Corti formation is the number that will be present in the mature tissue so that, in mice, the species most commonly used for studies of mammalian inner ear development, by embryonic day 18 (E18) 3 rows of OHC and a single row of IHC, are present and will remain until adulthood. However, it is worth noting that in the earliest stages of organ of Corti formation, but after cell cycle arrest has occurred, additional (supernumerary) hair cells can be generated; e.g. exposure of the early embryonic organ of Corti to retinoic acid results in the presence at E18 of up to 11 rows of OHC and 2 rows of IHC across the organ of Corti, with intervening supporting cells [23]. These cells arise in the absence of cell division; their cell fate has been altered. Normally, the cells from which the supernumerary hair and supporting cells derive would have gone on to be the nonsensory cells that border the sensory strip, and whilst the capacity to alter the fate of these cells is present only in the earliest stages of organ of Corti development – it is lost by E18 in mice – it indicates that these nonsensory cells in the mature organ of Corti are part of the same cell lineage from which hair cells and their immediately surrounding supporting cells arise. This may be important in the situation that may arise in people who have been deaf for some time whose organ of Corti is replaced by essentially a 'flat' epithelium derived from cells that may have the same 'genetic history' and potential as supporting cells.

REPAIR OF SENSORY EPITHELIA WITH HAIR CELL LOSS AND HAIR CELL REGENERATION

In all hair cell epithelia in all vertebrate classes that have been studied, the majority of conditions that cause death of hair cells do not affect supporting cells. Critically, when a

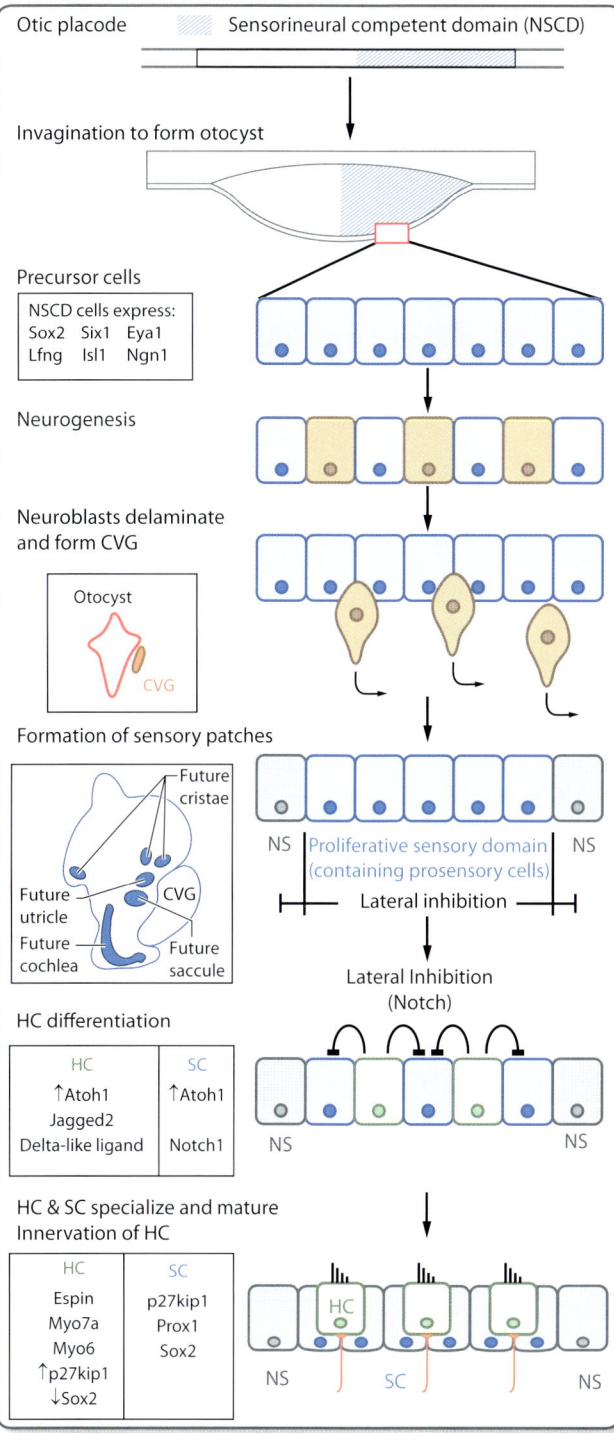

Figure 8.2 The otic placode invaginates to form the otocyst. In the ventral otocyst sensorineural competent domains (NSCD) form, containing the precursor cells for both neural and sensory cells. The precursor cells express various markers, including Sox2 and Ngn1. During neurogenesis, neuroblasts expressing Ngn1 and Delta1 are formed and then delaminate from the epithelium to form the cochleovestibular ganglion (CVG). The CVG gives rise to the spiral ganglion neurons that innervate hair cells. Following neuroblast delamination, the remaining prosensory cells form separate sensory patches in structures that will later become sensory organs – the three cristae of the semi-circular canals, the two maculae of the utricle and saccule, and the organ of Corti in the cochlea. Within the patches cells develop in a specific "salt and pepper" pattern by a process of lateral inhibition that is mediated by the Notch signalling pathway. As prosensory cells differentiate, Atoh1, a key transcription factor for hair cell differentiation, becomes upregulated in cells that will become hair cells, and these cells express Notch ligands (Jagged2 and Delta-like ligand) that inhibit the surrounding cells from becoming hair cells. Notch activation in the supporting cells promotes expression of Hes1 and Hes5 which inhibits Atoh1, preventing these cells from differentiating into hair cells. As the immature hair cells and supporting cells differentiate, they express a range of different genes and gene products some of which are indicated.

hair cell dies, the supporting cells are triggered to repair the epithelial lesion. The molecular mechanisms that initiate and regulate this important activity are unknown. At the epithelial surface, this can be observed as an expansion of the supporting cells to close any epithelial 'holes'. Recent live imaging work in the avian utricle has shown that this involves a rapid and coordinated response from the supporting cells, sealing up the epithelial surface using a purse-string like mechanism [24]. These data are in agreement with previous data from fixed specimens in mammalian tissue [25-27]. This repair response occurs sufficiently rapidly to maintain tissue integrity. In all non-mammalian vertebrates, new hair cells are then spontaneously regenerated from amongst the supporting cells.

Regeneration in nonmammalian vertebrates

Studies of birds (young chickens) exposed to loud sounds revealed that in the basilar papilla, the auditory epithelium, the noise-induced death of hair cells and their replacement by supporting cells is localised primarily to the frequency place along the cochlea of the damaging noise. Significant damage was observed 24 hours after onset of the noise exposure, but a few days after the exposure cells bearing small hair bundles with the characteristics of the normal immature hair cells were present, and within approximately 10 days the entire lesioned area had been replaced by new hair cells [28a]. Subsequent audiological assessments demonstrated functional recovery [28b]. A similar recovery of hair cells numbers (and of audition) after aminoglycoside-induced hair cell death in the basilar papilla [29] and in the vestibular sensory epithelia of birds [30,31] was subsequently observed. This work indicated the damage-induced regeneration of hair cells. The undamaged avian auditory epithelium does not produce new hair cells. However, it has been shown that avian vestibular organs continuously produce new hair cells throughout life [32,33] with hair cells dying and being replaced by new ones within a framework of almost constant total hair cell numbers. That hair cell regeneration occurs in the basilar papilla is of potential significance because just like mammals, birds are warm blooded, and also like mammals the number of hair cells in the basilar papilla is defined during embryonic development, and in the absence of any damage there is no subsequent addition of hair cells or cell division.

Initial analyses of the mechanisms of hair cell regeneration in the basilar papilla showed that the death of hair cells induced a reinitiation of cell division amongst the supporting cell population, with new hair cells (and supporting cells) arising from daughter cells of those divisions [34a, 34b]. Cell division was localised to the region of damage and continued only until hair cell numbers had recovered to the normal level and was then switched off. However, the factors regulating both the initiation and termination of cell division have not yet been identified. Some evidence of hair cell production outside the region of cell proliferation was also noted indicating a nonproliferative mode of regeneration [35,36]. Studies in the inner ears of newts in which hair cells had been ablated by aminoglycosides provided direct evidence for regenerating hair cells arising not as daughter cells of mitotic events but from a conversion of supporting cells into hair cells without intervening cell divisions [37]. It is now apparent that two mechanisms, nonmitotic 'transdifferentiation' or 'phenotypic conversion' of supporting cells into hair cells and mitotic regeneration, operate to regenerate hair cells. The two mechanisms are not mutually exclusive and in fact it appears that in the avian basilar papilla the first regenerated hair cells arise through phenotypic conversion, with hair cells (and possible replacement supporting cells) arising later following stimulation of supporting cell division [38,39]. However, it is also apparent that non-lethally damaged hair cells may have the capacity to repair; damaged hair cells may lose their hair bundles, withdraw their bodies into the body of the sensory epithelium, then re-emerge at the luminal surface and regrow their hair bundles [40]. Such a repair process could explain some of the functional recovery that has been observed [41]. This aspect of the recovery is potentially very important but is overlooked and understudied.

Repair and recovery of sensory epithelia after hair cell loss in mammals

Cell division does not occur in the mammalian inner ear following loss of hair cells in either the vestibular sensory epithelium or the organ of Corti. However, there is evidence for a limited capacity for endogenous or spontaneous hair cell regeneration in vivo in the mammalian vestibular organs [2,3,42-44]. Following ablation of hair cells after treatment of animals with aminoglycosides, supporting cells expand to fill the spaces once occupied by the hair cells. Cells bearing characteristic immature hair bundles are then apparent within 2 weeks of the end of the treatment. Hair cell numbers increase slowly over a period of about 8–12 weeks [2], but only a maximum of about one-third to one-half of the hair cells that are lost are replaced. These new hair cells appear to arise by phenotypic conversion of supporting cells [45].

In the organ of Corti, hair cell loss in most situations occurs progressively, usually beginning at the basal end, where high frequency sounds are detected, then spreading apically to affect cells responsible for detecting successively lower frequencies. OHC are damaged and lost first. IHC usually persist for some time and most commonly do not begin to disappear until after all OHC in their immediate neighbourhood have been lost. Loss of OHC results in loss of amplification, resulting in a 40–60 dB increase in the auditory threshold, equivalent to 'moderate' hearing loss. With loss of IHC, there is an inability to send messages to the brain, thus hearing impairment becomes severe to profound in the frequency regions affected. Following loss of IHC, afferent innervation disappears; mainly due to loss of the neurotrophic factors produced by the hair cells that are necessary for neuronal survival [21]. In the cochlear epithelium that remains after hair cell loss, Deiters' cells, the supporting cells that normally surround the OHC, repair and close the lesions and they maintain the cellular specialisations they acquired during the late stages of organ of Corti maturation: the phalangeal processes that provide structural support and connexins and other proteins (e.g. GLAST and KCC4) that are involved in maintaining homeostasis [46]. Our evidence suggests that the supporting cells do not appear to de-differentiate to a more immature status. Subsequently over longer periods however, the repaired organ of Corti may become reorganised. Nonsensory cells from outer, lateral side of the epithelium migrate across the Deiters' cell region and the pseudostratified columnar epithelium of the organ of Corti is replaced by a 'flat' epithelium of squamous-like cells covering the basilar membrane. During this reorganisation, the specialised supporting cells, the Deiters' cells and pillar cells, which normally are in contact with the hair cells, are lost. Such reorganisation is not always complete and can occur just in patches along the organ of Corti so that columnar and squamous-like regions are present in the same cochlea. Also the speed and extent of reorganisation appear to be dependent on genetic background [46]. These observations indicate that in a single 'profoundly deaf' cochlea there may be different types of epithelium along the organ of Corti, and that there may be differences between individuals in the cellular nature of the organ of Corti from which hair cells have been lost. These findings too have implications for any subsequent regenerative strategies.

The variable nature of the damaged or aged epithelium means that different regenerative approaches may be needed depending on what the pathology inside the cochlea is like. Thus, it will be critical to have excellent audiological assessment of this in any potential patients.

It is worth noting that recent work has indicated that subtle but important changes occur primarily at the level of the IHC synapses resulting in auditory deficits in the absence of hair cell loss [47,48]. This could still be a primary effect at the IHC itself since signalling to the synapse is critical for it regulation. Thus, further investigation of how trauma affects the IHCs themselves is still required.

These features of hair cell loss are of significance clinically for strategies aimed at regenerating cochlear hair cells and they raise such questions as: what is the patient group for which a regenerative strategy might be considered?; and what is the intended outcome of a regeneration strategy? With regard to the latter question, is a complete restoration of hair cells required, or simply restoration, principally, of IHC which might enhance neuronal cell survival thereby retaining the ability to detect auditory signals; or simply to restore some hair cells in the expectation that they will attract neurites from surviving spiral ganglion cells which may enhance the effectiveness of a cochlear implant?

Understanding the signals that regulate repair of the sensory epithelium

Ongoing research aimed at understanding the signalling mechanisms that regulate repair of the sensory epithelium when hair cells are lost is important since it could indicate potential therapeutic targets to stimulate a regenerative response in the organ of Corti. One such signalling mechanism is via the release of ATP that occurs when cells are damaged. Release of ATP triggers increases in intracellular Ca^{2+} in supporting cells that travel away from the damage site as intercellular waves [49-51]. In addition, faster damage-induced ATP-dependent intercellular Ca^{2+} waves have been also observed in hair cells [52]. The role of these Ca^{2+} waves are still under investigation, but they could be involved in activating the damage-induced response of supporting cells via the extracellular-signal-regulated kinases (ERK) pathway [51], a MAPK signalling pathway that is known to be important in cell proliferation, differentiation and migration. Activation of the ERK signalling pathway may well be important in determining the supporting cell repair response that allows phagocytic-like clearance of damaged hair cells [24,27, 52a, 52b] but further work is required to determine the nature of this role (see [53] for a more detailed review). Another important set of molecules that can regulate how tissue responds during damage are heat shock proteins (HSPs). These form a ubiquitous and conserved response to cellular stress (not only heat stress). In particular, HSP70 has been shown to be protective in aminoglycoside-induced hair cell loss in vitro and in vivo [54-56]. The upregulation of HSP70 occurs primarily in supporting cells [57] and again this indicates a critical involvement of those neighbouring cells in the survival and death of the hair cells. Heat shock is known to activate another mechanism within cells and that is the stress granule [58]. Recent work has indicated a potential role for this RNA-translation-regulation pathway in controlling how cochlear cells respond to damage [59]. The work described here would benefit from additional studies comparing such signalling mechanisms in mammals with those that are activated in nonmammalian vertebrates that exhibit hair cell regeneration. This could provide a greater understanding of how to stimulate endogenous regeneration in mammals.

STRATEGIES FOR REGENERATING HAIR CELLS IN THE MAMMALIAN EAR

Enhancing or triggering endogenous hair cell regeneration

One potential means to induce hair cell regeneration would be to trigger proliferation of cells in the organ of Corti through manipulation of the regulators of the cell cycle. Mice from which the gene encoding p27kip1, a cyclin-dependent kinase, has been deleted (p27kip1-null mice) show continued proliferation of supporting cells into adulthood and produce supernumerary hair cells [11,60]. It was suggested that the downregulation of p27kip1 may be critical in regulating the age-dependent proliferative capacity of mammalian cochlear supporting cells [61a]. However, the null mice were deaf and it is unclear how much the normal cellular development was affected by the absence of p27kip1. Conditional deletion of the gene using genetic techniques through which a gene can be normally expressed during development but 'switched off' in the adult showed that downregulation of p27kip1 in adult animals reinitiates cell division in the organ of Corti and vestibular sensory epithelia but does not appear to result in hair cell generation in undamaged tissues, i.e. ones with a normal complement of hair cells [61b]. Animals in which retinoblastoma protein (pRb), the cell cycle suppressor expressed by hair cells, is deleted by genetic manipulation show large numbers of hair cells to be generated by division of existing hair cells in the immature organ of Corti [19]. However, these hair cells begin to die fairly soon after their generation and when the deletion of pRb was targeted to the mature organ of Corti there was no proliferation [62a]. This finding attests to the possibility that the specialisations of cells in the organ of Corti that occur during late stages of maturation may also include a differentiation process that prevents induction of proliferation. The suggestion then is that some degree of cellular de-differentiation may be necessary for such approaches to work. Another important point to consider is that, although it may be possible to 'switch on' cell division, how to turn it off at the necessary point remains unknown. Obviously, any continued 'tumerous' proliferation in such a confined space as the cochlear duct would be disastrous for the organ.

An alternative strategy for endogenous regeneration of hair cells is to induce phenotypic conversion of supporting cells into hair cells. With such a strategy, as there is no proliferation, the number of supporting cells will decline unless the supporting cells can be replaced. This is the mechanism that occurs 'naturally,' although only to a limited extent in mammalian vestibular organs. Our greater understanding of how hair cells are produced and how their fate is determined has led to the use of Atoh1 (described earlier) as a therapy. In vivo viral infection or inoculation of Atoh1 into undamaged guinea pig ears resulted in 'ectopic' hair cells forming in the inner sulcus region of the organ of Corti and attracting neurites from the spiral ganglion [62b], suggesting the potential value of this strategy. Following this, the same group reported that when viral infection of Atoh1 was applied unilaterally to deafened guinea pigs, many infected cochlear supporting cells expressing Atoh1 were observed, a significant hair cell recovery was recorded and there was a recovery of auditory thresholds 8 weeks post-Atoh1 treatment when compared to the opposite ears (not inoculated with virus) of the same animals [63]. However, it is worth noting that this report still awaits replication by others. Other laboratories have been investigating the potential for Atoh1 viral therapy in mammalian vestibular organs in vivo after loss of hair cells caused by gentamicin. The authors describe a repopulation of the epithelium with hair cells at the same time as reduction in the number of supporting cells

[64,65]. This may suggest that enhancing phenotypic conversion in the vestibular organs where the cellular environment seems to be naturally conducive to this mode of hair cell regeneration is a more fertile prospect.

Another potential means to induce the phenotypic conversion of supporting cells in the mammalian inner ear is through inhibiting the 'Notch-Delta' pathway that suppresses differentiation of precursor cells as hair cells during normal development (see **Figure 8.2**). Whilst the genes involved in this pathway are downregulated as sensory epithelia mature, there is evidence that they are re-expressed during regeneration in chickens [66,67]. The Notch receptor is a transmembrane protein and when Delta proteins bind to it, the intracellular domain is cleaved away by a γ-secretase enzyme, and the intracellular fragment translocates to the nucleus to repress those genes that determine the hair cell fate, so specifying the cell as a supporting cell. There are a number of γ-secretase inhibitors, the most widely used being DAPT, which has been shown to result in cells that were destined to become nonsensory cells, adopting hair cell fates. In utricular maculae from adult mice maintained in culture and exposed to gentamicin to kill hair cells, incubation with DAPT leads to significant numbers of supporting cells beginning to express Atoh1 and then converting to cells that expressed hair cell markers and bearing immature hair bundles over a period of approximately 3 weeks [68]. Although the effect was primarily confined to a particular region of the macula, across the striola region, this study quite convincingly demonstrated the potential of the approach to induce enhancement of hair cell regeneration in the mammalian vestibular sensory epithelia. Subsequently, a similar strategy has been applied to the cochlea of adult animals in vivo using a more potent γ-secretase inhibitor (LY411575), applied unilaterally at the cochlear round window of cochlea of mice exposed to damaging noise levels. Three months after treatment and/or deafening, OHC numbers in the ear treated with the inhibitor were somewhat greater than those in the equivalent region of the opposite untreated ear where almost all hair cells were lost. There was no significant effect on the numbers of IHC. Auditory brainstem response (ABR) assessment of functional recovery showed a small but significant improvement in threshold predominantly in the 8–11 kHz region, reducing the hearing loss from 85 dB sound pressure level (SPL) to 75 dB SPL. It is hard to reconcile this effect with a recovery of OHC numbers and it is possible that the effect was primarily on the IHC to afferent nerve axis. The very modest response in the cochlea may be a further reflection of the difficulties of inducing hair cell regeneration in the adult organ of Corti even when the therapy is applied at the time of hair cell loss.

Endogenous stem or progenitor cells in the sensory epithelia of inner ear

Several studies have reported protocols for the isolation and differentiation in vitro of endogenous hair cell stem/progenitor cells from embryonic and neonatal rodents. Early protocols involved the dissociation of whole cochlear [69] or organ of Corti tissues [70], or automated sorting of cells based on fluorescent markers (fluorescence-activated cell sorting) in order to isolate supporting cell populations [61, 71-76].

Stem cells have a fundamental capacity for self-renewal. A widely used assay for potential stem cells is the ability to form spherical masses of cells in vitro and this has been used to isolate endogenous stem cells from many different tissues. Heller et al. isolated cells from mouse utricles that, using protocols that suppress endodermal and mesodermal fates and promote non-neural ectoderm, could be induced to form spheres in culture [77,78]. Sphere-forming cells could be obtained from the sensory epithelia of mouse utricles for up to at least 4 months postnatally, although the capacity was reduced compared to early postnatal stages. In the cochlea that capacity was much reduced after the first few postnatal and after 3 weeks was absent [78]. The otic progenitor cells were differentiated using serum-free medium with a defined growth factor differentiation medium to form cells that coexpressed the hair cell markers Atoh1, myosin VIIA (Myo7a), parvalbumin 3, and which showed voltage-dependent current recordings reminiscent of immature embryonic mouse hair cell activity. These markers are used along with others to indicate the cells as hair-cell-like cells (HCLCs).

Hu and Corwin [79] published the first protocol that produced hair cells entirely in vitro without the need for transplantation of cells into the ear of an embryo or coculture with other tissues. The starting cell population was cells isolated from embryonic chick sensory epithelia. The procedure involved the culture of these cells through multiple passages, after which the cells, having undergone an epithelial-to-mesenchymal transition, were reaggregated into spheres through suspension culture. These cell spheres developed HCLCs with hair bundles on the surface that formed a mosaic pattern alternating with other epithelial cells, reminiscent of the pattern seen in vivo. Electrophysiological methods were not used to assay for hair cell mechanotransduction, but testing with FM1-43 dye, that loads in to hair cells via the transduction channels [80] indicated that they were likely to be functional. Many of these differentiation procedures use sphere generation as an essential step in the differentiation protocols from rodent progenitor cells. Diensthuber et al. [81] characterised the different types of spheres that have been described in these reports, by dissociating embryonic mouse sensory epithelial cells and culturing these cells in suspension such that they became spheres. These were then differentiated in adherent culture to form HCLCs. Their work indicated that 'solid'-type spheres, rather than hollow spheres, gave the most HCLCs, consistent with other reports [78]. However, the HCLCs produced were only tested by immunocytochemistry for Atoh1, Myo7a and parvalbumin 3, with no indication of hair bundles specialisations or functional capability.

More recently, there has been significant interest in resident cells that express Lgr5, an orphan receptor of the Wnt signalling pathway proposed as a marker of stem/progenitor cells in the postnatal mouse cochlea. Lgr5-sorted cells have been cultured and can generate cells that show upregulation of hair cell markers Myo7a, parvalbumin 3 and calretinin [75,76]. It is early days for the Lgr5-positive cells but they may well prove to be an important source of cells for regenerative strategies.

Generating hair cells from stem cells

Steps toward generation of a mammalian hair cell epithelium in vitro (i.e. 'in a dish') have already been made. A stem cell-derived in vitro hair cell epithelium could provide an accessible source of large numbers of hair cells for biochemical studies and, for regenerative medicine, it could be used in drug screens for candidate molecules that could stimulate endogenous regeneration or for agents that might protect hair cells from ototoxicity or other forms of cellular damage. There is also the possibility for use in cell-based treatment for hair cell loss. The development of such a model also has the potential to reveal molecular mechanisms pertinent to hair cell development and regeneration.

A number of studies have reported protocols for the differentiation of HCLCs from embryonic stem cells (ESCs), induced pluripotent stem cells (iPSCs) or endogenous inner ear progenitor cells. Heller et al. [82] reported the first protocol that used mouse ESCs to generate inner ear progenitors in vitro. When transplanted into the embryonic chick ear, these progenitors were competent to respond to the environmental cues to integrate and differentiate into HCLCs in vivo. The same group further developed this protocol and generated ESC- and iPSC-derived HCLCs that showed morphological and physiological characteristics resembling immature hair cells [83]. The cells were positive for Myo7a and espin, which label the cell bodies and the actin-rich stereocilia bundles on the apical surface of hair cells respectively. The presence of hair bundles was confirmed by scanning electron microscopy from which hair bundle morphology could be observed, including the interstereociliary links, slanted asymmetric tops and tapered bases typical of hair cell stereocilia. Electrophysiological responses measured from mechanically stimulated hair bundles were consistent with evoked responses observed in immature hair cells.

The first effective use of human stem cells to generate otic cells came from Rivolta et al. who derived 'foetal auditory stem cells' from the embryonic cochleae of aborted fetuses and differentiated them into HCLCs in vitro [84]. In 2012, they adopted a similar protocol using human ESCs to again produce HCLCs (expressing markers Myo7a, Brn3c and Atoh1) in vitro [85]. The HCLCs did have apical projections that appeared to contain espin; although the structure of these projections was disorganised in comparison to a hair cell, it reflects some form of apical polarisation of the cells.

Much of the work on stem cells has required the use of feeder cells, cells cultured in the same dish as the stem cells producing or contributing important but unknown factors. For the generation of otic cells, the commonly used feeders are embryonic mouse periotic mesenchyme and chick utricle stromal cells. Although the use of mesenchymal feeder cells has been widespread, it appears that it is not essential for otic differentiation since HCLCs have been produced without the need for coculture or transplantation [76,81,85]. In addition, it has been reported that human ESCs were able to differentiate as HCLCs without the use of conditioned media or coculture. This could indicate that human cells might not require the stromal factors that the mouse cells do, or because the method of generating the otic progenitors was different and more inductive. However, the chick utricle stromal cells are still likely to be a source of the signal(s) that would allow the hair cells to mature more effectively.

Mesenchymal cells themselves are another potential source of stem cells for generating hair cells. Bone marrow-derived mesenchymal stem cells (BM-MSCs) or adipose-derived stem cells (ADSCs) are popular for their potential for clinical translation due to their ease of access, multipotent nature (ability to give rise to cells from more than one tissue) and lack of ethical controversy. BM-MSCs have been shown to be able, when induced appropriately, to express otic markers, including Atoh1, Brn3c, Sox2, Pax2, Pax8, Gata3 and Myo7a [86, 87].

Most recently, using mouse ESC cells Koehler et al. [88] have arguably defined a more successful protocol which produced HCLCs with the morphological and physiological characteristics of typical hair cells. In addition, it would seem that they have been able to recapitulate the development of a sensory epithelium and produce both hair cells and supporting cells. These studies indicate a great potential not only for generating useful in vitro hair cell epithelia but also for generating a source of implantable cells for regenerative medicine approaches. However, there is still much work to be done to see how any cellular-based therapies will be able to interact with a long since or even immediately damaged cochlear epithelium.

CONCLUSION

Currently, the possibility to regenerate cochlear hair cells as a therapy for deafness would still appear to be a distant prospect, but progress toward that goal has been made. The organ of Corti is highly and precisely organised and its complete restoration after hair cell loss will be difficult to achieve and reconnecting those cells to the appropriate neurons is also far from trivial. However, scattered or partial replacement of hair cells is not only more feasible but is also likely to improve the efficiency of cochlear implants; regenerated hair cells should produce the neurotrophins necessary for the survival of neurons and there is some experimental evidence that regenerated hair cells can attract neurites. If hair cells were regenerated on or close to the site of the original organ of Corti, neurites attracted from neurons remaining after loss of hair cells would be brought closer to the implant electrodes than would otherwise be the case, thereby improving efficiency. Although not covered by this review, another potential prospect is the possibility for direct restoration of the neurones themselves, perhaps derived from stem cells. This too would have positive impact for the use of cochlear implants. Regardless of the actual targets, approaches combining biological and technological interventions or therapies may be the way forward in restoring hearing.

However, the complications for hair cell regeneration in the organ of Corti are much less of an issue for vestibular sensory epithelia. The supporting cells of the vestibular sensory epithelia are not specialised in the same way as those of the organ of Corti; hair cell loss does not provoke such major changes in epithelial architecture in vestibular organs; and there appears to be some capacity for spontaneous hair cell regeneration in those epithelia. Thus, it will be much more straightforward to apply any proposed regenerative therapies to vestibular sensory tissues. If such therapies are successful, then they could also provide clues as to the conditions necessary for successful hair cell regeneration in the organ of Corti.

Key points for clinical practice

- Loss of and damage to hair cells in the organ of Corti is a major cause of hearing loss.
- Spontaneous regeneration of auditory hair cells does not occur in mammals, but is found in birds and reptiles.
- In noise-induced or age-related hearing loss, outer hair cells are lost initially, followed by inner hair cells (depending on the severity) and finally spiral ganglion cells. Thus different regenerative strategies may be needed depending the stage that a patient is in this process.
- Preliminary studies suggest that manipulating the expression of Atoh1 or inhibiting the Notch signalling pathway, can promote hair cell recovery.
- A promising approach to hair cell regeneration exploits embryonic stem cells. Stem cells injected into the cochlea can be made to differentiate into neurons and some recovery of function has been observed.
- Future work is essential in this area to understand the integration of replacement, regeneration and re-innervation of hair cells with the damaged cochlear epithelium, to enable the effective functional recovery of hearing.

REFERENCES

1. Rubel EW, Furrer SA, Stone JS. A brief history of hair cell regeneration research and speculations on the future. Hear Res 2013; 297:42–51.
2. Forge A, Li L, Nevill G. Hair cell recovery in the vestibular sensory epithelia of mature guinea pigs. J Comp Neurol 1998; 397:69–88.

3. Kawamoto KK, Izumikawa M, Beyer LA, Atkin GM, Raphael Y. Spontaneous hair cell regeneration in the mouse utricle following gentamicin ototoxicity. Hear Res 2009; 247:17–26.

4. Souter M, Nevill G, Forge A. Postnatal maturation of the organ of Corti in gerbils: morphology and physiological responses. J Comp Neurol 1997; 386:635–651.

5. Tolomeo JA, Holley MC. Mechanics of microtubule bundles in pillar cells from the inner ear. Biophys J 1997; 73:2241–2247.

6. Zetes DE, Tolomeo JA, Holley MC. Structure and mechanics of supporting cells in the guinea pig organ of Corti. PLoS One 2012; 7:e49338.

7. Boettger T, Hübner CA, Maier H, et al. Deafness and renal tubular acidosis in mice lacking the K-Cl co-transporter Kcc4. Nature 2002; 416:874–878.

8. Rozengurt N, Lopez I, Chiu CS, et al. Time course of inner ear degeneration and deafness in mice lacking the Kir4.1 potassium channel subunit. Hear Res 2003; 177:71–80.

9. Nickel R, Forge A. Gap junctions and connexins in the inner ear: their roles in homeostasis and deafness. Curr Opin Otolaryngol Head Neck Surg 2008; 16:452–457.

10. Ruben RJ. Development of the inner ear of the mouse: a radioautographic study of terminal mitoses. Acta Otolaryngol 1967;Suppl 220:1–44.

11. Chen P, Segil N. p27(Kip1) links cell proliferation to morphogenesis in the developing organ of Corti. Development 1999; 126:1581–1590.

12. Bermingham NA, Hassan BA, Price SD, et al. Math1: an essential gene for the generation of inner ear hair cells. Science 1999; 284:1837–1841.

13. Woods C, Montcouquiol M, Kelley MW. Math1 regulates development of the sensory epithelium in the mammalian cochlea. Nat Neurosci 2004; 7:1310–1318.

14. Zheng JL, Gao WQ. Overexpression of Math1 induces robust production of extra hair cells in postnatal rat inner ears. Nat Neurosci 2000; 3:580–586.

15. Adam J, Myat A, Le Roux I, et al. Cell fate choices and the expression of Notch, Delta and Serrate homologues in the chick inner ear: parallels with Drosophila sense-organ development. Development 1998; 125:4645–4654.

16. Daudet N, Lewis J. Two contrasting roles for Notch activity in chick inner ear development: specification of prosensory patches and lateral inhibition of hair-cell differentiation. Development 2005; 132:541–551.

17. Lang H, Fekete DM. Lineage analysis in the chicken inner ear shows differences in clonal dispersion for epithelial, neuronal, and mesenchymal cells. Dev Biol 2001; 234:120–137.

18. Fekete DM, Wu DK. Revisiting cell fate specification in the inner ear. Curr Opin Neurobiol 2002; 12:35–42.

19. Sage C, Huang M, Karimi K, et al. Proliferation of functional hair cells in vivo in the absence of the retinoblastoma protein. Science 2005; 307:1114–1118.

20. Sage C, Huang M, Vollrath MA, et al. Essential role of retinoblastoma protein in mammalian hair cell development and hearing. Proc Natl Acad Sci U S A 2006; 103:7345–7350.

21. Yang T, Kersigo J, Jahan I, Pan N, Fritzsch B. The molecular basis of making spiral ganglion neurons and connecting them to hair cells of the organ of Corti. Hear Res 2011; 278:21–33.

22. McKenzie E, Krupin A, Kelley MW. Cellular growth and rearrangement during the development of the mammalian organ of Corti. Dev Dyn 2004; 229:802–812.

23. Kelley MW, Xu XM, Wagner MA, Warchol ME, Corwin JT. The developing organ of Corti contains retinoic acid and forms supernumerary hair cells in response to exogenous retinoic acid in culture. Development 1993; 119:1041–1053.

24. Bird JE, Daudet N, Warchol ME, Gale JE. Supporting cells eliminate dying sensory hair cells to maintain epithelial integrity in the avian inner ear. J Neurosci 2010; 30:12545–12556.

25. Raphael Y, Altschuler RA. Scar formation after drug-induced cochlear insult. Hear Res 1991; 51:173–183.

26. Meiteles LZ, Raphael Y. Scar formation in the vestibular sensory epithelium after aminoglycoside toxicity. Hear Res 1994; 79:26–38.

27. Li L, Nevill G, Forge A. Two modes of hair cell loss from the vestibular sensory epithelia of the guinea pig inner ear. J Comp Neurol 1995; 355:405–417.

28a. Cotanche DA. Regeneration of hair cell stereociliary bundles in the chick cochlea following severe acoustic trauma. Hear Res 1987; 30:181–195.

28b. McFadden EA, Saunders JC. Recovery of auditory function following intense sound exposure in the neonatal chick. Hear Res 1989; 41:205–215.

29. Cruz RM, Lambert PR, Rubel EW. Light microscopic evidence of hair cell regeneration after gentamicin toxicity in chick cochlea. Arch Otolaryngol Head Neck Surg 1987; 113:1058–1062.

30. Weisleder P, Rubel EW. Hair cell regeneration in the avian vestibular epithelium. Exp Neurol 1992; 115:2–6.

31. Weisleder P, Rubel EW. Hair cell regeneration after streptomycin toxicity in the avian vestibular epithelium. J Comp Neurol 1993; 331:97–110.

32. Jørgensen JM, Mathiesen C. The avian inner ear. Continuous production of hair cells in vestibular sensory organs, but not in the auditory papilla. Die Naturwissenschaften 1988; 75:319–320.

33. Roberson DF, Weisleder P, Bohrer PS, Rubel EW. Ongoing production of sensory cells in the vestibular epithelium of the chick. Hearing Research 1992; 57:166–174.

34a. Corwin JT, Cotanche DA. Regeneration of sensory hair cells after acoustic trauma. Science 1988; 240:1772–1774.

34b. Ryals BM, Rubel EW. Hair cell regeneration after acoustic trauma in adult Coturnix quail. Science 1988; 240:1774–1776.

35. Adler HJ, Raphael Y. New hair cells arise from supporting cell conversion in the acoustically damaged chick inner ear. Neurosci Lett 1996; 205:17–20.

36. Roberson DW, Alosi JA, Cotanche DA. Direct transdifferentiation gives rise to the earliest new hair cells in regenerating avian auditory epithelium. J Neurosci Res 2004; 78:461–471.

37. Taylor RR, Forge A. Hair cell regeneration in sensory epithelia from the inner ear of a urodele amphibian. J Comp Neurol 2005; 484:105–120.

38. Cafaro J, Lee GS, Stone JS. Atoh1 expression defines activated progenitors and differentiating hair cells during avian hair cell regeneration. Dev Dyn 2007; 236:156–170.

39. Daudet N, Gibson R, Shang J, et al. Notch regulation of progenitor cell behavior in quiescent and regenerating auditory epithelium of mature birds. Dev Biol 2009; 326:86–100.

40. Gale JE, Meyers JR, Periasamy A, Corwin JT. Survival of bundleless hair cells and subsequent bundle replacement in the bullfrog's saccule. J Neurobiol 2002; 50:81–92.

41. Taura A, Kojima K, Ito J, Ohmori H. Recovery of hair cell function after damage induced by gentamicin in organ culture of rat vestibular maculae. Brain Res 2006; 1098:33–48.

42. Forge A, Li L, Corwin JT, Nevill G. Ultrastructural evidence for hair cell regeneration in the mammalian inner ear. Science 1993; 259:1616–1619.

43. Warchol ME, Lambert PR, Goldstein BJ, Forge A, Corwin JT. Regenerative proliferation in inner ear sensory epithelia from adult guinea pigs and humans. Science 1993; 259:1619–1622.

44. Lopez I, Honrubia V, Lee SC, et al. Quantification of the process of hair cell loss and recovery in the chinchilla crista ampullaris after gentamicin treatment. Int J Dev Neurosci 1997; 15:447–461.

45. Li L, Forge A. Morphological evidence for supporting cell to hair cell conversion in the mammalian utricular macula. Int J Dev Neurosci 1997; 15:433–446.

46. Taylor RR, Jagger DJ, Forge A. Defining the cellular environment in the organ of Corti following extensive hair cell loss: a basis for future sensory cell replacement in the Cochlea. PLoS One 2012; 7:e30577.

47. Kujawa SG, Liberman MC. Adding insult to injury: cochlear nerve degeneration after 'temporary' noise-induced hearing loss. J Neurosci 2009; 29:14077–14085.

48. Sergeyenko Y, Lall K, Liberman MC, Kujawa SG. Age-related cochlear synaptopathy: an early-onset contributor to auditory functional decline. J Neurosci 2013; 33:13686–13694.

49. Gale JE, Piazza V, Ciubotaru CD, Mammano F. A mechanism for sensing noise damage in the inner ear. Curr Biol 2004; 14:526–529.

50. Piazza V, Ciubotaru CD, Gale JE, Mammano F. Purinergic signalling and intercellular Ca2+ wave propagation in the organ of Corti. Cell Calcium 2007; 41:77–86.

51. Lahne M, Gale JE. Damage-induced activation of ERK1/2 in cochlear supporting cells is a hair cell death-promoting signal that depends on extracellular ATP and calcium. J Neurosci 2008; 28:4918–4928.

52a. Lahne M, Gale JE. Damage-induced cell-cell communication in different cochlear cell types via two distinct ATP-dependent Ca waves. Purinergic Signal 2010; 6:189–200.

52b. Abrashkin KA, Izumikawa M, Miyazawa T, et al. The fate of outer hair cells after acoustic or ototoxic insults. Hear Res 2006;218(1-2):20–29.

53. Monzack EL, Cunningham LL. Lead roles for supporting actors: critical functions of inner ear supporting cells. Hear Res 2013; 303:20–29.

54. Cunningham LL, Brandon CS. Heat shock inhibits both aminoglycoside- and cisplatin-induced sensory hair cell death. JARO 2006; 7:299–307.

55. Taleb M, Brandon CS, Lee FS, et al. Hsp70 inhibits aminoglycoside-induced hair cell death and is necessary for the protective effect of heat shock. JARO 2008;9:277–289.

56. Taleb M, Brandon CS, Lee FS, et al. Hsp70 inhibits aminoglycoside-induced hearing loss and cochlear hair cell death. Cell Stress Chaperones 2009; 14:427–437.

57. May LA, Kramarenko II, Brandon CS, et al. Inner ear supporting cells protect hair cells by secreting HSP70. J Clin Invest 2013; 123:3577–3587.
58. Anderson P, Kedersha N. RNA granules. J Cell Biol 2006; 172:803–880.
59. Towers ER, Kelly JJ, Sud R, Gale JE, Dawson SJ. Caprin-1 is a target of the deafness gene Pou4f3 and is recruited to stress granules in cochlear hair cells in response to ototoxic damage. J Cell Sci 2011; 124:1145–1155.
60. Löwenheim H, Furness DN, Kil J, et al. Gene disruption of p27(Kip1) allows cell proliferation in the postnatal and adult organ of Corti. Proc Natl Acad Sci U S A 1999; 96:4084–4088.
61a.White PM, Doetzlhofer A, Lee YS, Groves AK, Segil N. Mammalian cochlear supporting cells can divide and trans-differentiate into hair cells. Nature 2006; 441:984–987.
61b.Oesterle EC, Chien WM, Campbell S, Nellimarla P, Fero ML. p27(Kip1) is required to maintain proliferative quiescence in the adult cochlea and pituitary. Cell Cycle 2011; 10:1237–1248.
62a.Weber T, Corbett MK, Chow LM, et al. Rapid cell-cycle reentry and cell death after acute inactivation of the retinoblastoma gene product in postnatal cochlear hair cells. Proc Natl Acad Sci USA 2008; 105:781–785.
62b.Kawamoto K, Ishimoto S, Minoda R, Brough DE, Raphael Y. Math1 gene transfer generates new cochlear hair cells in mature guinea pigs in vivo. J Neurosci 2003;23(11):4395–400.
63. Izumikawa M, Minoda R, Kawamoto K, et al. Auditory hair cell replacement and hearing improvement by Atoh1 gene therapy in deaf mammals. Nat Med 2005; 11:271–276.
64. Staecker H, Praetorius M, Baker K, Brough DE. Vestibular hair cell regeneration and restoration of balance function induced by math1 gene transfer. Otol Neurotol 2007; 28:223–231.
65. Kraft S, Hsu C, Brough DE, Staecker H. Atoh1 induces auditory hair cell recovery in mice after ototoxic injury. Laryngoscope 2013; 123:992–999.
66. Hawkins RD, Bashiardes S, Powder KE, et al. Large scale gene expression profiles of regenerating inner ear sensory epithelia. PLoS One 2007; 2:e525.
67. Ku YC, Renaud NA, Veile RA, et al. The transcriptome of utricle hair cell regeneration in the avian inner ear. J Neurosci 2014; 34:3523–3535.
68. Lin V, Golub JS, Nguyen TB, et al. Inhibition of Notch activity promotes nonmitotic regeneration of hair cells in the adult mouse utricles. J Neurosci 2011; 31:15329–15339.
69. Doetzlhofer A, White PM, Johnson JE, Segil N, Groves AK. In vitro growth and differentiation of mammalian sensory hair cell progenitors: a requirement for EGF and periotic mesenchyme. Dev Biol 2004; 272:432–447.
70. Malgrange B, Belachew S, Thiry M, et al. Proliferative generation of mammalian auditory hair cells in culture. Mechs Dev 2002; 112:79–88.
71. Zhai Shi L, Wang BE, Zheng G, et al. Isolation and culture of hair cell progenitors from postnatal rat cochleae. J Neurobiol 2005; 65:282–293.
72. Savary E, Hugnot JP, Chassigneux Y, et al. Distinct population of hair cell progenitors can be isolated from the postnatal mouse cochlea using side population analysis. Stem Cells 2007; 25:332–339.
73. Zhang Y, Zhai SQ, Shou J, et al. 'Isolation, growth and differentiation of hair cell progenitors from the newborn rat cochlear greater epithelial ridge. J Neurosci Methods 2007; 164:271–279.
74. Sinkkonen ST, Chai R, Jan TA, et al. Intrinsic regenerative potential of murine cochlear supporting cells. Sci Rep 2011; 1:26.
75. Chai R, Kuo B, Wang T, et al. Wnt signaling induces proliferation of sensory precursors in the postnatal mouse cochlea. Proc Natl Acad Sci U S A 2012; 109:8167–8172.
76. Shi F, Kempfle JS, Edge AS. Wnt-responsive Lgr5-expressing stem cells are hair cell progenitors in the cochlea. J Neurosci 2012; 32:9639–9648.
77. Li H, Liu H, Heller S. Pluripotent stem cells from the adult mouse inner ear. Nature Med 2003a; 9:1293–1299.
78. Oshima K, Grimm CM, Corrales CE, et al. Differential distribution of stem cells in the auditory and vestibular organs of the inner ear. JARO 2007; 8:18–31.
79. Hu Z, Corwin JT. Inner ear hair cells produced in vitro by a mesenchymal-to-epithelial transition. Proc Natl Acad Sci U S A 2007; 104:16675–16680.
80. Gale J E, Marcotti W, Kennedy HJ, Kros CJ, Richardson GP. FM1-43 dye behaves as a permeant blocker of the hair-cell mechanotransducer channel. J Neurosci 2001; 21:7013–7025.
81. Diensthuber M, Oshima K, Heller S. Stem/progenitor cells derived from the cochlear sensory epithelium give rise to spheres with distinct morphologies and features. JARO 2009; 10:173–190.
82. Li H, Roblin G, Liu H, Heller S. Generation of hair cells by stepwise differentiation of embryonic stem cells. Proc Natl Acad Sci USA 2003b; 100:13495–13500.

83. Oshima K, Shin K, Diensthuber M, Peng AW, Ricci AJ, Heller S. Mechanosensitive hair cell-like cells from embryonic and induced pluripotent stem cells. Cell 2010; 141:704–716.

84. Chen W, Johnson SL, Marcotti W, et al. Human fetal auditory stem cells can be expanded in vitro and differentiate into functional auditory neurons and hair cell-like cells. Stem Cells 2009; 27:1196–1204.

85. Chen W, Jongkamonwiwat N, Abbas L, et al. Restoration of auditory evoked responses by human ES-cell-derived otic progenitors. Nature 2012; 490:278–282.

86. Boddy SL, Chen W, Romero-Guevara R, et al. Inner ear progenitor cells can be generated in vitro from human bone marrow mesenchymal stem cells. Regenerative Med 2012; 7:757–767.

87. Durán Alonso MB, Feijoo-Redondo A, Conde de Felipe M, et al. Generation of inner ear sensory cells from bone marrow-derived human mesenchymal stem cells. Regenerative Med 2012; 7:769–783.

88. Koehler KR, Mikosz AM, Molosh AI, Patel D, Hashino E. Generation of inner ear sensory epithelia from pluripotent stem cells in 3D culture. Nature 2013; 500:217-221.

Chapter 9

Vestibular implants

Richard F Lewis, Daniel M Merfeld

INTRODUCTION

The vestibular labyrinth in the inner ear senses angular and linear head motion and the orientation of the head relative to gravity. This information is used by the brain to generate eye movements that keep images stationary on the retina during head motion (the vestibulo-ocular reflex or VOR), and contributes to the perception of head motion and orientation and to postural control. When the vestibular labyrinth is damaged, patients experience impaired vision during head movements, abnormal percepts of motion and orientation, and imbalance. Since the hair cells in the labyrinth do not spontaneously regenerate, peripheral vestibular damage is usually permanent. Vestibular damage is caused by a large variety of aetiologies, including head trauma, viral infection of the labyrinth or vestibular nerve, ototoxic drugs, Ménière's disease and numerous other disorders. People with substantial vestibular damage have difficulty with balance, particularly in the dark, during head turns, and whilst standing on compliant or moving surfaces and have impaired vision when the head is motion, with illusionary movement of the visual world (oscillopsia) caused by image motion on the retina. Since the currently available treatments are generally inadequate to significantly improve these symptoms, over the past 15 years increasing interest has focused on the development and implementation of vestibular prosthetics to treat severe vestibular damage. Analogous to cochlear implants for people with severe hearing loss, vestibular implants utilise sensors (i.e., motion sensors) to transduce the information normally sensed by the vestibular labyrinth and provide this information to the brain by electrically stimulating the afferent nerves that innervate the labyrinthine end-organs.

The vestibular labyrinth (**Figure 9.1**) consists of three semicircular canals and two otolith organs (see [1] for a review). The three semicircular canals in each ear are mutually perpendicular, and the canals in the two ears are paired anatomically and functionally. The lateral canals, one per ear, form one pair, as do the anterior canal and posterior canals in opposite ears. The afferent nerves innervating the canals discharge at a tonic rate of about 100 spikes/s when the head is stationary. When the head rotates, the cupula in the canal is deflected and this modulates activity in the hair cells that are embedded

Richard F Lewis MD, Department of Otology and Laryngology, Harvard Medical School; Jenks Vestibular Physiology Laboratory, Boston, USA.

Daniel M Merfeld PhD, Harvard Medical School, Department of Otology and Laryngology; Jenks Vestibular Physiology Laboratory, Boston, USA. Email: dan_merfeld@meei.harvard.edu (for correspondence)

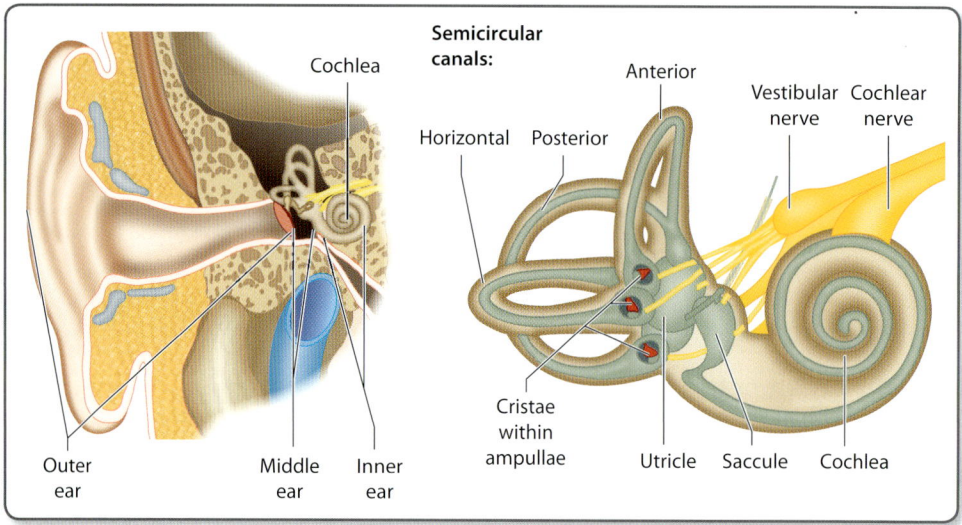

Figure 9.1 The panel shows an isolated view of the vestibular labyrinth. Prominent in this figure are the fluid filled loops that define the semicircular canals. One can also see each semicircular canal's crista, located in an expansion of each canal called the ampulla. These cristae are the transduction sites and are innervated by the afferent neurons as illustrated. Also shown are the cochlear as well as the utricle and saccule, which represent the vestibular system's otolith organs. Reproduced with permission from Wolfe JM, Kluender KR, Levi DM, et al. Sensation and perception. Sunderland, MA: Sinauer Associates; 2012.

in the cupula. All hair cells in each canal are oriented in the same direction such that deflections in one direction reduce their activity (thereby reducing the discharge rates in that canal's ampullary neurons) and deflections in the opposite direction increase activity (leading to an increased discharge rates in those same ampullary neurons). The modulation in discharge rate in each ampullary nerve is proportional to angular head velocity perpendicular to the plane of the canal. Furthermore, each pair of canals functions in a 'push-pull' manner such that head rotations that increase the discharge rate from one canal decrease it in the paired canal in the other ear. For example, rotations towards the left increase the rate of discharge from the left lateral canal and decrease the rate from the right lateral canal. Given these anatomic and physiologic features, it is apparent that semicircular canal function could be simulated by an implant in a fairly straightforward manner: angular head velocity in the plane of a given canal is measured and this velocity signal is used to modulate the strength of electrical stimulation applied to that canal's ampullary nerve, depending on the direction of the head rotation. With this approach, an implant could provide the brain with a reasonable facsimile of the angular head velocity signal that is normally provided by the semicircular canal.

The otolith organs consist of the saccule and utricle. With the head upright, the saccule is oriented near earth-vertical and the utricle is near earth-horizontal. The otolith organs transduce the vector sum of gravity and the inertial force produced by linear acceleration. Unlike the canals, the polarities of the hair cells in the otolith organs are organised in a complex, radial manner, and reverse their direction near the centre. Because of this complex organisation, when an otolith organ is stimulated by linear acceleration or a change in head orientation, hair cell modulation is not uniform but rather varies substantially depending on the cells' otolithic maculae location. This complex pattern cannot be simulated by an implant by simply modulating the strength of electrical stimulation applied to the otolith organ's afferent nerve. For this, reason, vestibular implants have so far focused on the semicircular canals, with the goal of providing a signal to the brain that encodes angular head velocity in three dimensions in a reasonably physiologic manner.

Below we summarise the progress made to date in the development and testing of a canal implant. Firstly we will review the technological developments that have occurred over the past 15 years, and then will review the behavioural experiments that have tested how well the brain can use the signals provided by the implant to generate the eye movement, perceptual and postural responses that are normally mediated by the vestibular system.

TECHNOLOGICAL DEVELOPMENT

The semicircular canal implant was originally conceptualised by Merfeld and Gong [2,3] and subsequent technical improvements have been refinements of this approach. We will therefore first describe the 'prototype' canal prosthesis as it was originally devised, and will then review the subsequent technical developments.

Prototype canal implant

The prototype prosthesis consists of an angular velocity sensor that is used to measure angular head velocity about one rotational axis, an electrode implanted in one canal near the ampulla and the circuitry and power needed to use the angular velocity signal to calculate and provide electrical stimulation to the implanted electrode. Since the canals are high-pass filters (e.g. they respond well to high-frequency rotations and poorly to low-frequency rotations), the angular head velocity signal was high-pass filter with a cut-off frequency of 0.03 Hz, simulating the frequency dependence of the normal canal, and this filtered angular head velocity was used to determine the rate of electrical stimulation. To provide bidirectional motion cues to the brain using an implant in one ear, the prototype prosthesis provided a tonic rate of electrical stimulation that was well above the normal baseline firing rate of the canal afferent nerves. Conceptually, it was hypothesised that the brain would adapt to the imbalance in vestibular tone produced by an artificially increased tonic firing rate in one ear, and that stimulation could then modulate up or down to signal the direction of the head rotation. This approach could therefore provide the brain with information about head rotations both towards and away from the implanted ear. The tonic stimulation rate was chosen to be 200 or 250 pulses per sec (pps), well above the resting discharge rate of canal afferents [1] and this stimulation rate modulated up or down based on a hyperbolic tangent transfer function that related the filtered angular head velocity to the rate of electrical stimulation. The hyperbolic tangent function was chosen because it allows the rate of stimulation to modulate in a nearly linear fashion over a large part of the physiologic range of angular head velocities but saturates at the extremes of this physiologic range. The basic unit of stimulation was the biphasic, charge-balance current pulse. The amplitude of the pulses was determined during the initial electrode 'tuning' but then remained constant, and the head motion was encoded by changes in the rate that these pulses were applied to the ampullary nerve, similar to the manner in which canals normally encode angular head velocity. The electrodes used in the early experiments were insulated wires with the tip stripped, with the return site inserted in the ipsilateral temporalis muscle. In sum, the prototype implant measured angular head velocity about one rotational axis with a small rate sensor, this signal was high-pass filter to simulate normal canal dynamics and the filtered head velocity signal was used to modulate the rate of biphasic current pulses supplied to an electrode implant in one canal near the ampulla.

Electrode development

The early experiments were performed with an electrode with one stimulation site at its tip and a return in a relatively distant location. Two problems were associated with this approach. Firstly, the ability to effectively stimulate the canal ampullary nerve proved to be highly dependent on the precise location of the stimulation site in the canal, so very small movements of the electrode tip during surgical insertion or subsequently would markedly alter stimulation efficacy. Secondly, since the return electrode was relatively remote, the current path was not highly constrained so current spread often occurred, and this could produce significant electrical stimulation of the afferent nerves of the other canals or the facial nerve. These problems were largely overcome by introducing electrodes with multiple sites [4,5]. Since multiple stimulation and return sites are available on these electrodes, during electrode tuning the optimal combination of stimulation and return sites could be determined, which would produce the largest eye movements in the plane of the instrumented canal but would not significantly activate the afferent innervation of the other canals or the facial nerve. Multisite electrodes therefore allowed much improved control over the site of pulse delivery and the current path between the stimulation and return sites.

Multidimensional implant

As described above, the prototype implant measured angular head velocity about one rotational axis and provided electrical stimulation to one canal's afferent nerve. For almost all early experiments, the sensitive axis of the velocity sensor was aligned with that of the lateral canals and the electrode was implanted in one lateral canal [6,7]. A logical extension of this approach was to use three angular velocity sensors, each of which has its sensitive axis aligned with one of the three canals, and to provide electrical stimulation to all three canals by implanting electrodes near each canal's ampullary nerve. With this approach, the prosthesis senses angular head velocity in three dimensions and encodes this velocity vector by modulating the stimulation rate of three implanted electrodes, with the change in stimulation rate in each canals' electrode dependent on the component of the angular velocity that is aligned with that canals' velocity sensor [8,9].

Optimising electrical stimulation

Controlling the axis

Ideally, the three-dimensional angular velocity of the head should be encoded in the three canal ampullary nerves in a manner which lacks any 'cross-talk' between nerves. For example, if the head rotates about an axis aligned with the lateral canal's sensitive axis, only the afferents innervating the lateral canal should modulate their rate of discharge. The most straightforward way to assess how well the head rotation is encoded in this manner is to compare the rotational axis of the head to that of the eyes (e.g. the VOR). These axes should be perfectly aligned, as they are when the VOR is generated by the normal labyrinth.

In contrast, the prosthesis generally does not produce a VOR response with an axis that is perfectly aligned with the axis of head rotation [7]. Despite the use of multisite electrodes to constrict the extent of current flow, this is almost certainly because the electrical stimulation provided in one canal does spread to activate the afferent nerves innervating other canals to some degree. This problem can be efficiently solved in the prosthesis software; however, if the rotational axis of the eye produced by each of the three implanted electrodes is measured in isolation, then stimulation of two or three electrodes is combined to closely align the axis of eye rotation with the axis of head rotation [10]. The prosthesis software can therefore correct the rotational axis of the signal provided by the prosthesis by providing modulation in more than one electrode for any head rotation, an approach that recapitulates the mechanisms used by the brain to optimise the VOR's rotational axis.

Increasing the dynamic range of the prosthesis

The dynamic range over which the canal afferents can be stimulated is limited by two factors. There is an upper limit to their firing rate which is approximately 450 Hz, so stimulating electrically at frequencies higher than this will not yield neurons firing at these higher rates of stimulation. There is also a lower limit to the rate of stimulation, since the afferents normally discharge spontaneously at a rate of about 100 Hz. If the electrical stimulation is lowered below the normal tonic rate of afferent firing, these neurons will not decrease their firing rate below their normal spontaneous level. There is no known way to increase the upper limit of the rate of afferent firing, but if one could reduce the spontaneous rate of firing, then it would be feasible to modulate the rate of afferent firing below 100 Hz, thereby extending the dynamic range downward. Recent work suggests that the tonic rate of activity can be reduced by employing direct current stimulation in a charge-balanced fashion, and this approach could therefore potentially increase the dynamic range of the canal prosthesis [11].

Improving information transfer from the prosthesis to the ampullary nerve

The canals use rate coding to provide the brain with information about the angular velocity of the head, as changes in firing rate in the primary afferent are proportional to the angular velocity of the head. The prototype canal prosthesis and most of the subsequent prosthesis iterations have similarly encoded angular head velocity using the rate of current pulses supplied to the electrode, not in the amplitude of the current pulses. There is no a priori reason; however, why a prosthesis must emulate normal physiology, and it is clear from the earliest studies that VOR responses could be generated by modulating either the rate or amplitude (current) of the pulses [2]. Recent work has demonstrated that when both the rate and amplitude of the pulses are modulated in tandem, there is a significant nonlinear interaction between these two parameters, as the eye movements evoked with this approach are substantially larger than those produced by a simple sum of the rate and amplitude effects [12]. Comodulation of pulse rate and amplitude may therefore be a useful way to increase the ability of the prosthesis to generate larger amplitude VOR responses, although this approach has not yet been used with any form of chronic stimulation. Therefore, it is not clear that the amplification of the eye movement response with comodulation is indicative of an improvement in the transfer of information from the prosthesis to the ampullary nerve. Nor is it clear how well the brain can adapt to such comodulation.

BEHAVIOURAL EXPERIMENTS

Almost all of the behavioural experiments to date have focused on measuring VOR responses during either acute or chronic electrical stimulation of the canal ampullary nerves, and almost all of these experiments have been performed in animals. Below we will review the most salient features of these experiments, focusing on adaptation to the tone imbalance produced by the high resting rate of prosthetic stimulation, and evidence that the VOR generated by the prosthesis interacts in a qualitatively normal manner with otolith cues and undergoes relatively normal adaptation during chronic stimulation. More recent studies examining tilt perception and postural control in nonhuman primates and eye movements and posture in humans during acute stimulation will also be briefly reviewed.

Tone adaptation – resolution of spontaneous nystagmus

Normally the spontaneous activity in the ampullary nerves is very closely matched between the two ears [1]. When this baseline tone becomes imbalanced, as occurs when a high tonic stimulation rate drives the afferents to fire at higher baseline rate on one side, the clearest behavioural consequence is spontaneous nystagmus, and in humans this is known to be associated with the subjective sensation of rotation (e.g. vertigo). Whilst tonic stimulation at a rate of 200 or 250 Hz in one ear does cause a brisk spontaneous nystagmus, this nystagmus attenuates fairly rapidly and is usually gone within 24 hours [13]. Several experiments in guinea pigs have evaluated how the nystagmus response is affected by repeatedly turning stimulation on and off [13], or by ramping the rate of stimulation up slowly over many hours [14]. In the former case, the nystagmus became much smaller with repetitive transitions between the stimulation-on and stimulation-off states, which could represent habituation or dual-state adaptation that allows the animal to minimise nystagmus with the stimulation on or off (**Figure 9.2**).

Experiments which slowly ramped up the stimulation rate suggested that both of these mechanisms are most likely contributory, and also showed that a high tonic rate of stimulation can be reached without a meaningful nystagmus response if the stimulation rate is increased gradually over hours [14]. These results could be used to guide the rate that stimulation is turned on and off in human subjects so that vertigo symptoms are minimised, and this approach could also potentially be useful to abort acute vertigo attacks due to Ménière's and similar diseases that cause symptoms by sudden changes in tone balance [15].

Interaction between multiple stimulated canals – evidence for linearity

A basic assumption of a multidimensional prosthesis (or a bilateral prosthesis in one or more dimensions) is that the effects of each electrode's stimulation are independent of each other and that they sum linearly. This presumption was tested most thoroughly in squirrel monkeys with electrodes in each lateral canal. This study demonstrated quantitatively that the eye movement responses resulting from bilateral lateral canal stimulation are very nearly the same as the sum of each electrode's individual effect [16]. This observation is fundamental to the implementation of bilateral prosthetic stimulation, and for prosthetics that stimulate multiple canals within the same ear [10].

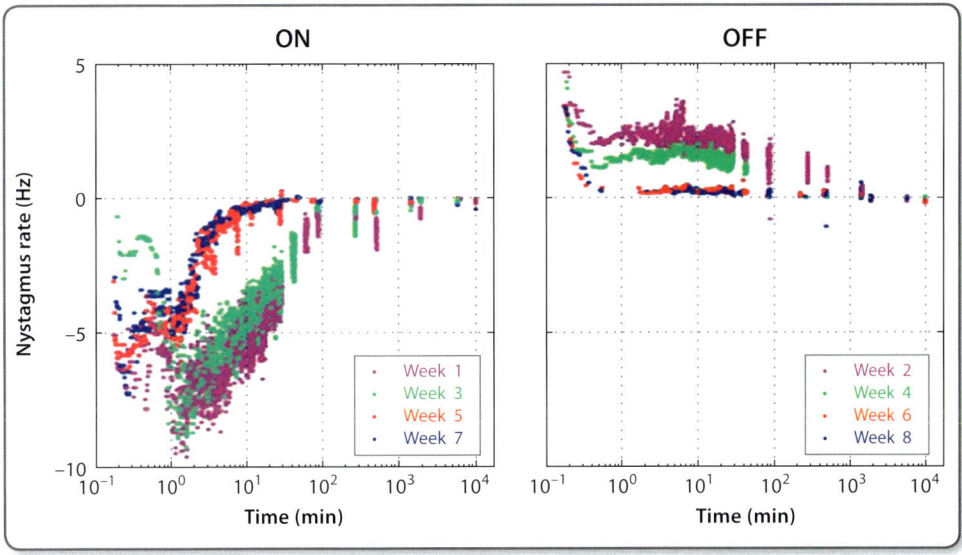

Figure 9.2 Horizontal quick phases plotted versus time (on a logarithmic scale), showing the rate of quick phases when tonic electrical stimulation was turned on repeatedly (weeks 1, 3, 5 and 7) and then off after a week of continuous stimulation (weeks 2, 4, 6 and 8). During repeated on/off cycles, the quick phase rate declined, both when the stimulation was turned and when it was turned off. Reproduced with permission from Merfeld et al. [13].

Vestibulo-ocular reflex – interaction between the implant stimulation and other sensory cues

The signal carried by the canal ampullary nerve during implant stimulation is quite different from the natural firing of the canal's primary afferent nerve. Whilst single unit recordings of peripheral afferents during stimulation are not yet available, recordings in the vestibular nuclei during implant stimulation have demonstrated an abnormally high degree of synchrony in the timing of neuronal discharge [17]. Because of this and other nonphysiologic features of the implant-mediated canal afferent signal, it was not known if the brain could utilise this implant stimulation in a physiologic manner. More specifically, rotational signals carried by the canal afferents normally interact with the gravitoinertial cues provided by the otolith organs, and they interact with visual signals that guide adaptation of the VOR. Both of these elements are critical to the success of a canal prosthesis. The 'canal–otolith' interaction is a fundamental aspect of central vestibular processing, as it is considered to be the mechanism used by the brain to estimate head orientation relative to gravity and to discriminate head tilts from translation. The use of visual cues to drive VOR adaptation is critical because the VOR produced by the prosthesis will never have perfect gain and axis characteristics, and like the normal VOR, it is presumed that central adaptive mechanisms will need to be engaged by the implant to optimise the kinematic features of the VOR.

Interaction between implant stimulation and otolith signals

The effects of otolith inputs on the rotational signals provided by the canals are most readily studied by measuring how head tilt affects the angular VOR. In normal subjects, if the head is tilted whilst a canal rotational signal is present, the VOR response is attenuated ('dumping') and its rotational axis shifts to align with gravity ('spatial orientation') [1]. Both of these effects are mediated by the velocity storage integrator in the brain, which is a critical element of normal central vestibular function. We studied if the prosthetic canal input interacts with gravity in a similar manner by stimulating one lateral canal whilst an animal was upright or tilted in roll. We found that qualitatively similar dumping and spatial orientation effects occurred when the angular velocity signal was provided by prosthetic input and in the normal animal (**Figure 9.3**) [18]. These observations demonstrate that the brain can synthesise the prosthetic signal with otolith-mediated gravitational cues, and furthermore, that the velocity storage network in the brain can be engaged by the prosthetic canal input.

Adaption of the VOR during chronic implant stimulation

The principal characteristics of the VOR are their amplitude (gain), their phase and axis relative to the head motion and their symmetry. Our experiments in squirrel monkeys [6,7] are the only long-term studies of prosthetic stimulation to date, as the animals' VOR responses were measured during unilateral lateral canal prosthetic stimulation for periods up to 1 year. We found that when the head was rotated in the plane of the lateral canal, a compensatory horizontal VOR response was elicited which reduced image motion on the retina. Each time the implant was turned on, the VOR gain initially dropped [7] presumably because of habituation or other mechanisms that reduced the peripheral or central sensitivity to the electrical stimulus. Over time, however, the VOR gain gradually increased, showing that VOR gain adaptation was occurring. The two-dimensional axis of the eye rotation also improved over time, as did the symmetry of the VOR. The VOR phase showed an abnormally large phase lead for low frequencies of rotation that did not change during the long period of stimulation [7]. These results show that visual signals can be used

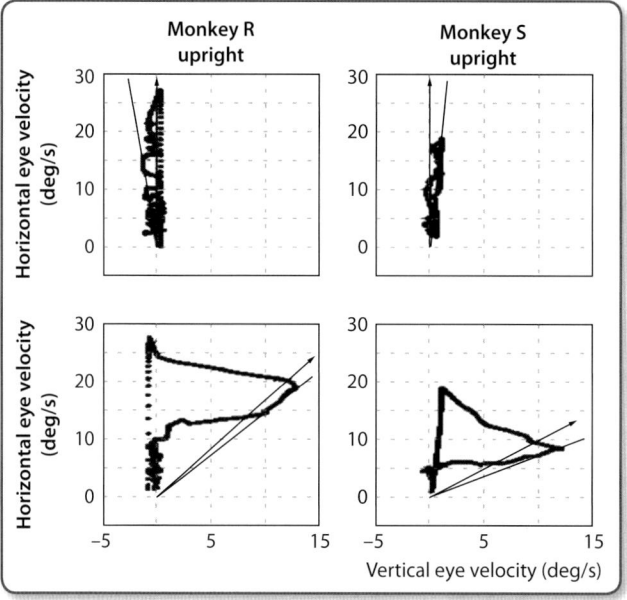

Figure 9.3 Eye movements produced by electrical stimulation of one lateral canal with the animal upright or tilted 45° in the roll plane. When the monkeys were upright, the eye velocity was almost entirely horizontal and the rotational axis was closely aligned with gravity (arrow). When the monkeys were tilted, however, the otolith signal interacted with the electrically induced lateral canal signal such that a substantial vertical component also developed and shifted the eye's rotational axis towards the direction of gravity (arrow).

by the brain to improve the gain, axis and symmetry of the VOR. Similar axis adaptation has also been demonstrated in rhesus monkeys using a three-dimensional prosthesis over a time frame of a week [19]. A more dramatic example of axis adaptation occurred in an experiment where we dissociated the plane of the angular velocity sensor and the stimulated canal. We aligned the velocity sensor with the lateral canals, but the stimulating electrode was in the posterior canal, so yaw head rotations produced vertical and torsional eye movements. Over a week of stimulation the VOR rotational axis shifted substantially towards the compensatory direction, as the vertical and torsional VOR responses produced by yaw rotation declined whilst the horizontal response increased [20].

Perceptual and postural studies in nonhuman primates

As outlined above, there is substantial evidence that a canal prosthesis can produce VOR responses that reduce retinal image motion, interact with otolith signals and undergo adaptation guided by visual feedback. The vestibular system is also important for the perception of head orientation and motion, and for postural control. Indeed, patients with vestibular disorders are primarily affected by abnormal perceptions (e.g. vertigo) and by ataxia, whilst visual symptoms related to an impaired VOR (e.g. oscillopsia) are often less bothersome. There is therefore a clear dichotomy between the vestibular-mediated behaviour that has been most thoroughly studied (the VOR) and the behaviours that are most significant to patients with vestibular dysfunction. For this reason, we began to study the effects of the canal prosthesis on the perception of head orientation and postural control in rhesus monkeys.

Perception of head orientation

We trained monkeys to perform a subjective visual vertical (SVV) task, where they learn to rotate a light bar so that is parallel to gravity, and then tested them on this task in the presence and absence of unilateral posterior canal electrical stimulation. We found that the stimulation produced shifts in SVV responses that were consistent with a misperception of roll tilt of the head towards the stimulated canal (**Figure 9.4**) [21]. These results provide the first evidence that the perception of head orientation can be modulated by electrical stimulation of a canal. We subsequently measured SVV responses during dynamic roll tilt over a frequency range of 0.005–0.4 Hz in the normal monkey, after severe bilateral vestibular ablation was introduced, and during three-dimensional prosthetic stimulation of the canals in one ear in the ablated animal. Preliminary results demonstrate that the perception of head orientation is accurate during roll tilt in the normal monkey, that it is degraded substantially after vestibular ablation and that it improves when prosthetic stimulation is provided to the ablated animal [22,23].

Postural control

Vestibular signals are thought to contribute to postural control primarily by providing the brain with an accurate estimate of head orientation relative to gravity, which is combined with information encoding head orientation relative to the body to produce an internal estimate of body orientation relative to gravity [24]. Since our perceptual studies suggest that the first step of this process (encoding of head orientation relative to gravity) is improved by prosthetic stimulation in vestibulopathic subjects, a reasonable assumption is that it would similarly improve postural control. Vestibulopathic patients have more pronounced problems with balance during quiet stance when visual and proprioceptive

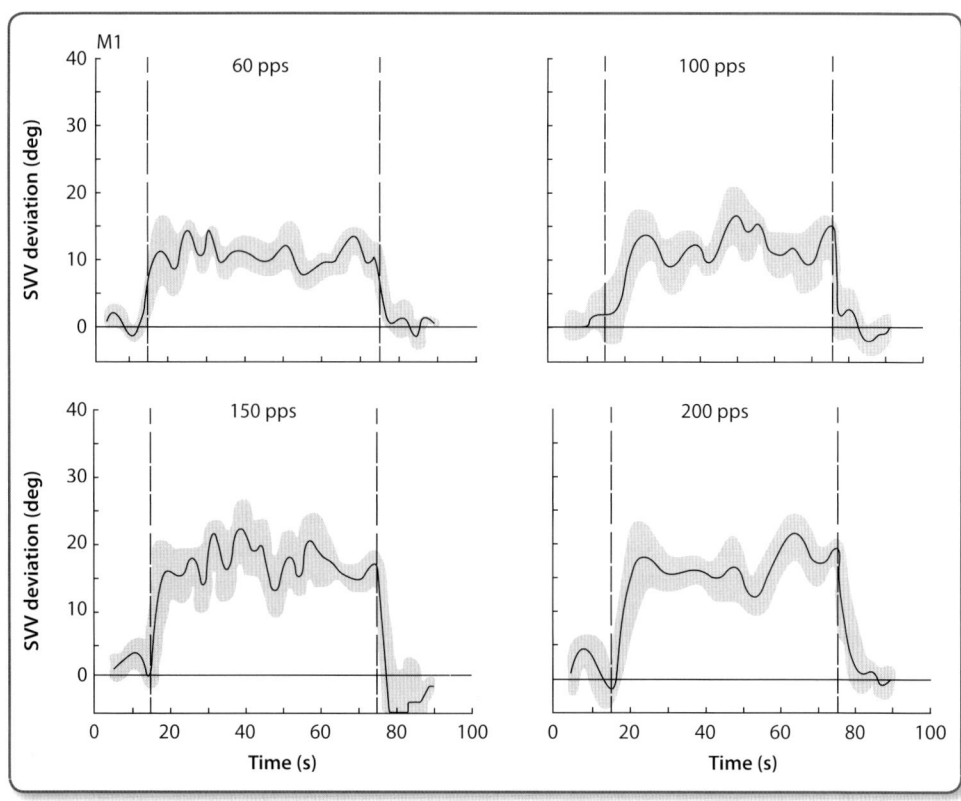

Figure 9.4 Deviation of the subjective visual vertical (SVV, y axis) versus time, before, during and after electrical stimulation of one posterior canal. The period of stimulation is marked by the vertical lines, and during that interval the SVV responses shifted away from the stimulated ear, consistent with a misperception of head tilt towards the ear receiving the stimulation. Reproduced with permission from Lewis et al. [18].

cues are minimised, during rotation of the support surface and during head turns [1,24]. We therefore developed protocols to measure postural control in rhesus monkeys during each of these behaviours in the normal and ablated states and studied the effect of prosthetic stimulation during quiet stance and in response to head turns. Preliminary results indicate that postural stability in vestibulopathic animals was not improved during quiet stance when prosthetic stimulation was provided, even if visual and proprioceptive cues were minimised. Conversely, we found that postural stability during head turns did improve in vestibulopathic monkeys when the prosthesis was activated [22,23]. These results suggest that a canal prosthesis can improve postural control, but it may be primarily useful in situations when angular head velocities are relatively high, such as during head turns.

HUMAN STUDIES

Prosthetic studies in humans have been quite limited to date, and have explored eye movement and postural responses during acute electrical activation of the canal ampullary nerves. Eye movements that approximate the plane of the activated canal have been generated with acute electrical canal stimulation [25] suggesting that similar to results in animal studies, a VOR will be elicitable in humans during motion-modulated electrical stimulation. Postural sway in a direction that approximates the orientation of the electrically stimulated canal has also recently been reported in human subjects, which demonstrates that postural responses in humans can also be modified with selective activation of individual canals [26].

CONCLUSION AND FUTURE DIRECTIONS

This chapter reviewed the substantial advances made towards the implementation of a three-dimensional semicircular canal prosthesis in human subjects. Whilst many elements regarding the optimal approach to transfer angular velocity information to the brain via electrical stimulation of canal ampullary nerves remain to be worked out, it seems likely that devices similar to those currently being studied in nonhuman primates will be used for the initial human studies, and that over time these devices will be serially refined. One important aspect of vestibular implants, which will require substantial additional study, is their safety, both in the acute postimplantation period and during chronic stimulation that may have durations measured in years or even decades. Preliminary studies indicate that the prosthesis electrodes can be implanted in animal or human canals without significantly reducing the function remaining in the implanted canal [27]. Furthermore, hearing appears to be largely preserved after electrodes are implanted in the canals [27,28]. These results suggest that human subjects most likely will not suffer additional vestibular or auditory deficits following implantation of a canal prosthesis. Despite this, the most appropriate initial human subjects will almost certainly be those with little residual vestibular or auditory function, to minimise the possibility that additional damage will be incurred by electrode implantation. It may be most feasible to initially couple vestibular implantation to cochlear implant surgery in deaf subjects, which would require these studies to focus on subjects with minimal vestibular and auditory function in both ears.

The effects of chronic implantation and stimulation could relate to mechanical changes due to electrode insertion in the canal, such as fibrotic or bony growths around the electrode, which could reduce both the efficacy of electrical stimulation and of the canal's residual function. Very little pathology is currently available that focuses on vestibular implants in this regard. We published temporal bone pathology in squirrel monkeys that did not demonstrate osseous changes around the electrode [7], even though these have been described with cochlear implants. In addition, chronic high-frequency electrical stimulation could have reversible or irreversible effects on the peripheral and central vestibular systems. Since stimulation is charge balanced and is provided at rates in the physiologic range, it seems unlikely that large numbers of primary afferents or secondary neurons will be damaged by chronic stimulation, although such effects have been described in the auditory system [29]. It appears more likely that changes in the neural component of the vestibular system will be functional and reversible. For example, the reduction in sensitivity to stimulation that was inferred by the rapid drop in VOR gain when stimulation was begun, and the abnormally high degree of synchrony in the firing of neurons in the vestibular nuclei, could both have substantial and detrimental effects on the ability of the prosthesis to engender effective long-term activation of the central vestibular circuitry. Future work will need to assess these effects more fully and to develop methods to obviate them. For example, very high (e.g. 5 kHz) stimulation [30] that is superimposed on the motion-modulated prosthetic signal may be effective in desynchronising activity in primary and secondary vestibular neurons, which would more closely simulate normal neural activity and perhaps would produce in parallel improved behavioural responses.

In conclusion, enormous progress has been made in the past 15 years in the field of vestibular implants, and a solid foundation now exists to further develop this field in both animal models and human subjects. The ultimate efficacy of this approach in patients with severe vestibular deficits remains to be determined, however, and numerous advances will be needed to move this field forward with the hope that vestibular implants may someday mirror the success of cochlear implants.

Key points for clinical practice

- Peripheral vestibular damage is a common and disabling problem.
- Treatment at present is limited to physical therapy which aims to maximise the brain's compensation to the peripheral damage.
- Over the past decade significant advances have been made in the development of a canal implant that provides the brain with information about the angular velocity of the head.
- The implant has been shown to generate a compensatory vestibulo-ocular that reduces retinal image motion during head movements, which would reduce the oscillopsia experienced by patients with severe vestibular hypofunction during head movements.
- Less is known about the ability of a canal implant to improve perception of motion and orientation or postural control, but preliminary results from rhesus monkeys suggest that these effects are feasible, and data from humans shows a canal implant can impact posture.
- Current goals are to optimise the manner in which the implant conveys information about angular head motion to the brain and to translate the implant to appropriate human subjects.

REFERENCES

1. Liberman MC, Rosowski JJ, Lewis RF. Physiology and pathophysiology. In: Merchant SN and Nadol JB (eds), Shucknect's pathology of the ear. Hamilton, ON: BC Decker; 2010.
2. Gong W, Merfeld DM. Prototype neural semicircular canal prosthesis using patterned electrical stimulation. Ann Biomed Eng 2000; 28:572–581.
3. Gong W, Merfeld DM. System design and performance of a unilateral horizontal semicircular canal prosthesis. IEEE Trans Biomed Eng 2002; 49:175–181.
4. Valentin NS, Hageman KN, Dai C, Della Santina CC, Fridman GY. Development of a multichannel vestibular prosthesis prototype by modification of a commercially available cochlear implant. IEEE Trans Neural Syst Rehabil Eng 2013; 21:830–839.
5. Nie K, Ling L, Bierer SM, Kaneko CR, et al. An experimental vestibular neural prosthesis: design and preliminary results with rhesus monkeys stimulated with modulated pulses. IEEE Trans Biomed Eng 2013; 60:1685–1692.
6. Merfeld DM, Haburcakova C, Gong W, Lewis RF. Chronic vestibule-ocular reflexes evoked by a vestibular prosthesis. IEEE Trans Biomed Eng 2007; 54:1005–1015.
7. Lewis RF, Haburcakova C, Gong W, Makary C, Merfeld DM. Vestibuloocular reflex adaptation investigated with chronic motion-modulated electrical stimulation of semicircular canal afferents. J Neurophysiol 2010; 103:1066–1079.
8. Dai C, Fridman GY, Davidovics NS, et al. Restoration of 3D vestibular sensation in rhesus monkeys using a multichannel vestibular prosthesis. Hear Res 2011; 281:74–83.

9. Chiang B, Fridman GY, Dai C, Rahman MA, Della Santina CC. Design and performance of a multichannel vestibular prosthesis that restores semicircular canal sensation in rhesus monkey. IEEE Trans Neural Syst Rehabil Eng 2011; 19:588–598.

10. Davidovics NS, Rahman MA, Dai C, et al. Multichannel vestibular prosthesis employing modulation of pulse rate and current with alignment precompensation elicits improved VOR performance in monkeys. J Assoc Res Otolaryngol 2013; 14:233–248.

11. Fridman GY, Della Santina CC. Safe direct current stimulation to expand capabilities of neural prostheses. IEEE Trans Neural Syst Rehabil Eng 2013; 21:319–328.

12. Davidovics NS, Fridman GY, Della Santina CC. Co-modulation of stimulus rate and current from elevated baselines expands head motion encoding range of the vestibular prosthesis. Exp Brain Res 2012; 218:389–400.

13. Merfeld DM, Gong W, Morrissey J, et al. Acclimation to chronic constant-rate peripheral stimulation provided by a vestibular prosthesis. IEEE Trans Biomed Eng 2006; 53:2362–2372.

14. Lewis RF, Nicoucar K, Gong W, Haburcakova C, Merfeld DM. Adaptation of vestibular tone studied with electrical stimulation of semicircular canal afferents. J Assoc Res Otolaryngol 2013; 14:331–340.

15. Wall C 3rd, Merfeld DM, Rauch SD, Black FO. Vestibular prostheses: the engineering and biomedical issues. J Vestib Res 2002-2003; 12:95–113.

16. Gong W, Haburcakova C, Merfeld DM. Vestibulo-ocular responses evoked via bilateral electrical stimulation of the lateral semicircular canals. IEEE Trans Biomed Eng 2008; 55:2608–2619.

17. Mitchell DE, Della Santina CC, Cullen KE. Characterization of central vestibular neuron responses during electrical stimulation delivered by a vestibular prosthesis. Abstr Soc Neurosci 2013; 265.02.

18. Lewis RF, Haburcakova C, Gong W, Karmali F, Merfeld DM. Spatial and temporal properties of eye movements produced by electrical stimulation of semicircular canal afferents. J Neurophysiol 2012; 108:1511–1520.

19. Dai C, Fridman GY, Chiang B, et al. Directional plasticity rapidly improves 3D vestibule-ocular reflex alignment in monkeys using a multichannel vestibular prosthesis. J Assoc Res Otolaryngol 2013; 14:863–877.

20. Lewis RF, Gong W, Ramsey M, et al. Vestibular adaptation studied with a prosthetic semicircular canal. J Vestib Res 2002-2003; 12:87–94.

21. Lewis RF, Haburcakova C, Gong W, Lee D, Merfeld D. Electrical stimulation of semicircular canal afferents affects the perception of head orientation. J Neurosci 2013; 33:9530–9535.

22. Thompson LA, Haburcakova C, Gong W, et al. Responses evoked by a vestibular implant providing chronic stimulation. J Vestib Res 2012; 22:11–15.

23. Lewis RF, Haburcakova C, Gong W, et al. Vestibular prosthesis tested in rhesus monkeys. Conf Proc IEEE Eng Med Biol Soc 2011; 2011:2277–2279.

24. Stapley PJ, Ting LH, Kuifu C, Everaert DG, Macpherson JM. Bilateral vestibular loss leads to active destabilization of balance during voluntary head turns in the standing cat. J Neurophysiol 2006; 95:3783–3797.

25. Guinand N, Guyot JP, KIngma H, Kos I, Pelizzone M. Vestibular implants: the first steps in humans. Conf Proc IEEE Eng Med Biol Soc 2011; 2011:2262–2264.

26. Philips C, Defrancisci C, Ling L, et al. Postural responses to electrical stimulation of the vestibular end organs in human subjects. Exp Brain Res 2013; 229:181–195.

27. Rubinstein JT, Bierer S, Kaneko C, et al. Implantation of the semicircular canals with preservation of hearing and rotational sensitivity: a vestibular neurostimulator suitable for clinical research. Otol Neurotol 2012; 33:789–796.

28. Tang S, Melvin TA, Della Santina CC. Effects of semicircular canal electrode implantation on hearing in chinchillas. Acta Otolaryngol 2009; 129:481–486.

29. Shepard RK, Clark GM. Effect of high electrical stimulation intensities on the auditory nerve using brain stem response audiometry. Ann Otol Rhinol Laryngol Suppl 1987; 128:50–52.

30. Rubinstein JT, Wilson BS, Finley CC, Abbas PJ. Pseudospontaneous activity: stochastic independence of auditory nerve fibers with electrical stimulation. Hear Res 1999; 127:108–118.

Chapter 10

The medical treatment of vascular anomalies

Oren Cavel, Julie Powell, Josée Dubois, Patrick Froehlich

INTRODUCTION

The correct understanding and use of terminology when describing a vascular anomaly is important for its proper management, as well as for allowing interinstitutional collaboration in research and guideline elaboration (**Table 10.1**). Vascular anomalies are divided into vascular tumours and vascular malformations, the latter further divided into either slow-flow (venous, lymphatic and capillary) or fast-flow (arteriovenous malformations and fistulas). As indicated by their names, vascular tumours or neoplasms result from abnormal cellular division and growth usually involving the endothelial layer, whereas vascular malformations have an inactive endothelium and probably represent a localised anomalous development in utero.

The clinical course of these two groups of lesions is also quite distinctive. Vascular tumours can be present at birth (congenital haemangioma – CH) or appear during infancy (infantile haemangioma – IH) or childhood, and can have a typical evolution phase as well as, depending on their type, an involution phase (IH and rapidly involuting CH). Vascular malformations, on the other hand, usually show a commensurate growth with the child or a slow progression and never regress.

Systemic and local pharmacotherapy exists for some vascular tumours (**Table 10.2**), but its use for vascular malformations is still experimental. Embolisation or sclerotherapy (**Table 10.3**) are usually used in the treatment of the latter group, whereas surgery and laser therapy can be helpful for both categories of lesions. This chapter describes the treatment of vascular lesions by systemic or local administration of drugs and by sclerotherapy. Embolisation, surgical treatment, and the use of laser are not detailed.

Oren Cavel MD, Department of Otorhinolaryngology, Sainte-Justine University Hospital, University of Montreal, Quebec, Canada
Email: orencavel@gmail.com (for correspondence)

Julie Powell MD, Director, Pediatric Dermatology, Associate Clinical Professor, Department of Dermatology, Sainte-Justine University Hospital, University of Montreal, Quebec, Canada

Josée Dubois MD MSc FRCPC, Department of Radiology, Sainte-Justine University Hospital, University of Montreal, Quebec, Canada

Patrick Froehlich MD PhD, Department of Otolaryngology, Sainte-Justine University Hospital, University of Montreal, Quebec, Canada

Table 10.1 Updated International Society for the Study of Vascular Anomalies (ISSVA) classification system	
Vascular tumours	**Vascular malformations**
Infantile haemangioma	Slow flow: Lymphatic malformation Venous malformation Capillary malformation
Congenital haemangioma (CH): Rapidly involuting CH Noninvoluting CH	
	Fast flow: Arterial malformations Arteriovenous malformation or fistula
Tufted angioma	
Haemangioendothelioma	Complex combined malformations
Adapted from [1]	

Table 10.2 Summary of main agents used in IH therapy			
	Advantages	**Drawbacks**	**Dose (range)**
Propranolol	Rapid and significant response No upper age limit	Only 5 years experience for this indication Rare risk of hypoglycemia, bradycardia and hypotension	2 mg/kg/day (1–3 mg/kg/day)
	Acetabulol – possibly less insomnia Nadolol – longer half life than propranolol, no blood brain barrier crossing		
	Timolol – local application, no systemic side effects		
Steroids	40 years experience as the former gold standard Useful in complex cardio-cerebro-vascular anomalies (ex- PHACE syndrome)	Frequent steroid side effects, short term Effective in proliferative phase only Less effective than propranolol	3 mg/kg/day (2–4 mg/kg/day)

Table 10.3 Summary of main agents used for LM sclerotherapy			
	Principal use	**Advantages**	**Disadvantages**
OK 432	Macrocystic LMs	Very low toxicity	Limited availability
Doxycycline	Macrocystic and microcystic LMs	Availability, low toxicity within therapeutic range	Rarely: hypoglycaemia, metabolic acidosis and haemolytic anaemia
Bleomycin	Microcystic LMs, sensitive regions	Seems the most efficient for microcysts, can be directly infiltrated into the lesion, produces less swelling	Theoretic risk of pulmonary fibrosis with high cumulative dose
LM, lymphatic malformation.			

VASCULAR TUMOURS

Infantile haemangioma

Whilst 90% of all IHs do not cause significant disturbance and can be left alone to proliferate and involute without intervention, it is often not the case for those located at the head and neck.

The indications for treatment are as follows:

- Airway obstruction
- Functional impairment in periorificial or orbital lesions
- Aesthetic and psychological consideration
- Ulcerated tumours
- Lesions at risk, as a segmental type that bares more complications and has a poorer outcome

Those classical indications might expand, as the balance between aesthetic considerations and drug-associated risks is shifting with the use of propranolol.

BETA-BLOCKERS

Propranolol

Five years after the first report of its use in the treatment of IH, propranolol has been widely adopted as the first-line treatment in many institutions [2,3]. The observation of its dramatic effect on IH size and colour (**Figures 10.1** and 10.**2**), along with its availability in paediatric hospitals and the relatively safe profile of its use, made it particularly appealing to physicians. Numerous case series were published describing a rate of positive response to propranolol above 90% [4,5], and a recent national multicentre review [6] that included 1130 patients found that resistance to propranolol occurred in only 0.9% of the cases. However, the degree of involution was quantified in fewer than 10 articles.

The only published prospective study comparing propranolol to another treatment was by Hogeling et al. [7], who reported on a randomised, double-blind, placebo-controlled trial enrolling 40 children. They found that after 24 weeks of treatment there was a 60% decrease in the IH volume in the propranolol group compared to 14% in the placebo group, in addition to a significant improvement in the tumours' redness and elevation on investigator scores from clinical photographs.

Two studies [8,9], analysing >20 patients each, provided a retrospective comparison to steroidal treatment and found the treatment with propranolol to be superior both in efficacy and the occurrence of side effects. In one of those studies, by Bertrand et al., the researchers deduced by matching patients treated with either propranolol or steroids according to the type, location, size and patient's age. In addition, two meta-analyses on the effectiveness of propranolol in the treatment of IH of either the airway [10] or a nonspecified location [11] found that the reported success rates with propranolol were far superior to the success rates with any other treatment, including steroids, laser and vincristine.

Propranolol treatment was also reported to be associated with a shorter time to pain control and healing of ulcerated IHs [5,12], although other contributing factors such as analgesic medication and wound dressing are hard to isolate and a comparison to other

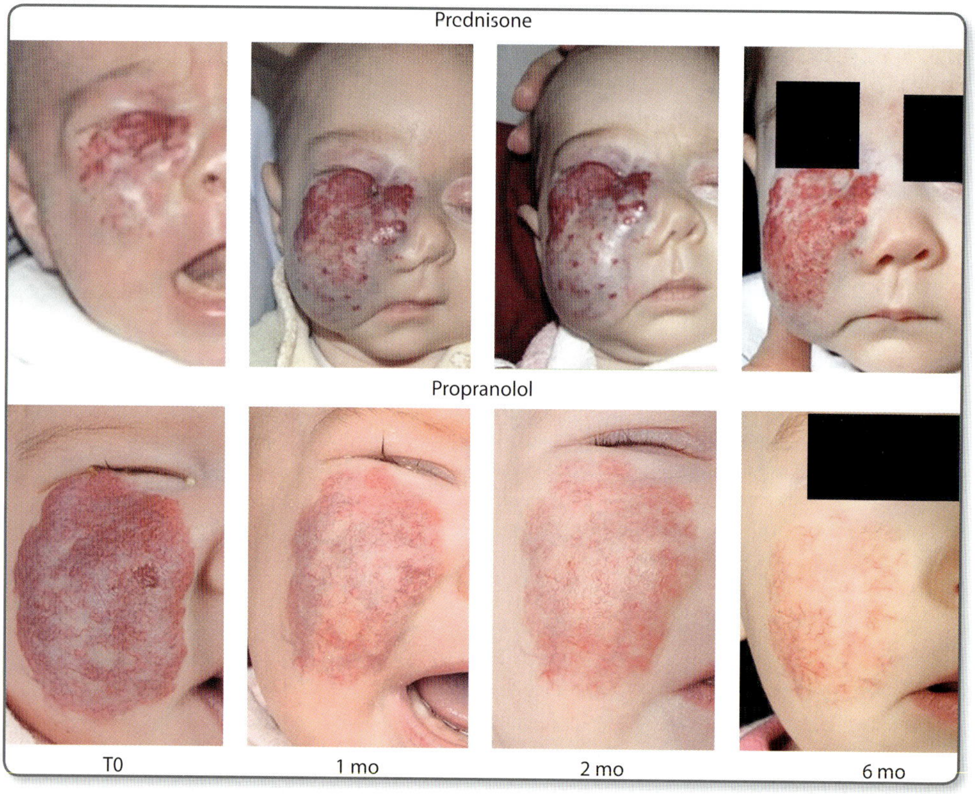

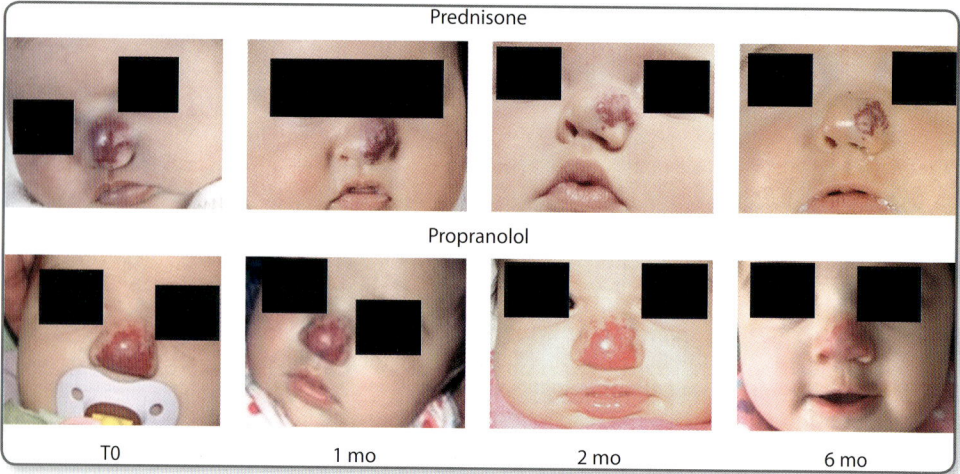

Figure 10.1 Response to prednisone (upper row) or propranolol (lower row) treatment in two patients with cheek IH involving the lower eye lid.

Figure 10.2 Response to prednisone (upper row) or propranolol (lower row) treatment in two patients with IH involving the nasal tip.

drugs was not made. Interestingly, ulcers sometimes appear in segmental IHs under propranolol treatment that could, theoretically, be attributed to a massive drug-induced apoptosis.

Propranolol is a nonselective blocker of the β-adrenergic receptor. It inhibits nor/epinephrine-mediated sympathetic actions and thus produces a negative inotropic and chronotropic effect on the heart, an inhibition of the release of renin in the kidney and a decrease in glycogenolysis in the liver and muscle. Seventy-five per cent of oral propranolol is eliminated by a first-pass metabolism in the liver, and the remaining 25% achieve peak plasma levels 1–3 hours after ingestion. Its metabolism involves cytochrome P450, which means an increase in bioavailability in the case of hepatic impairment or a competing drug.

The mechanism of action of propranolol on IH is still under research, and different theories have been suggested to clarify it, including capillary vasoconstriction associated with a change in colour and texture, inhibition of angiogenesis by reducing vascular endothelial growth factor (VEGF) levels [13], inhibition of matrix metalloproteinase expression and the renin–angiotensin axis [14], and an increase in apoptosis. Interestingly, one report describes a case [15] of acute 'rebound' increase in the size of a subglottic IH put on b-mimetic drugs for cardiac surgery, after an initial good response to propranolol for >6 months. However, one can propose alternative explanations, such as consequences of the surgery or the endotracheal intubation.

Dose

The usual dose of propranolol is 2 mg/kg per day divided to two to three times daily oral dosing [2,16]. It is recommended to start from 1 mg/kg per day or a lower dose and increase it gradually to avoid a significant cardiac response. The final dose can be individualised according to the patient's IH response, generally in the range of 1–3 mg/kg per day, but possibly up to 5 mg/kg. When a steroidal treatment is simultaneously administered (see steroid section below), the dose of propranolol is not altered.

Initial monitoring

Before the initiation of treatment with propranolol, a cardiovascular examination is performed, supplemented by an electrocardiogram if necessary. Basic monitoring of healthy children should include the measurement of blood pressure and heart rate 1 and 2 hours after the ingestion of the first one to three doses and again after each dose escalation. Suggested criteria for starting in an inpatient setting include airway lesion, corrected age under 8–10 weeks, comorbidity and inadequate familial support [16].

Measurement of response

The initial response of IH to propranolol is usually rapid, appearing right after the first doses, in the form of a softening of the mass and a decrease in its blushing, or as a decrease in wheezing and dyspnoea for airway lesions. Follow-up should include serial photographs of apparent IH taken according to the same parameters, or an endoscopy in the case of airway lesions. Many qualitative and a few quantitative ways to assess the effect can be found in the literature, including visual analogue scales, volume calculation on imaging, ultrasound (US) measurement of tumour volume and flow Doppler vessel density [17] or the use of a new haemangioma assessment scale [18].

Duration of treatment

A study providing evidence for the optimal duration of treatment has not yet been published. In most institutions, the treatment is continued for 6–12 months, as its cessation before the age of 10–12 months, i.e. during the natural proliferative phase, poses a greater risk of regrowth. In such cases, propranolol treatment is resumed and is usually effective. There is no clear age limit to the use of propranolol, as partial response is observed when the drug is initiated at an age corresponding to the involution phase [4] (**Figure 10.3**), or even later.

Contraindications

All the conditions listed below are relative contraindications, where treatment benefit should be weighed against risk:

- Cardiovascular – sinus bradycardia, hypotension, heart block greater than first degree, heart failure
- Asthma
- PHACE syndrome (see below)

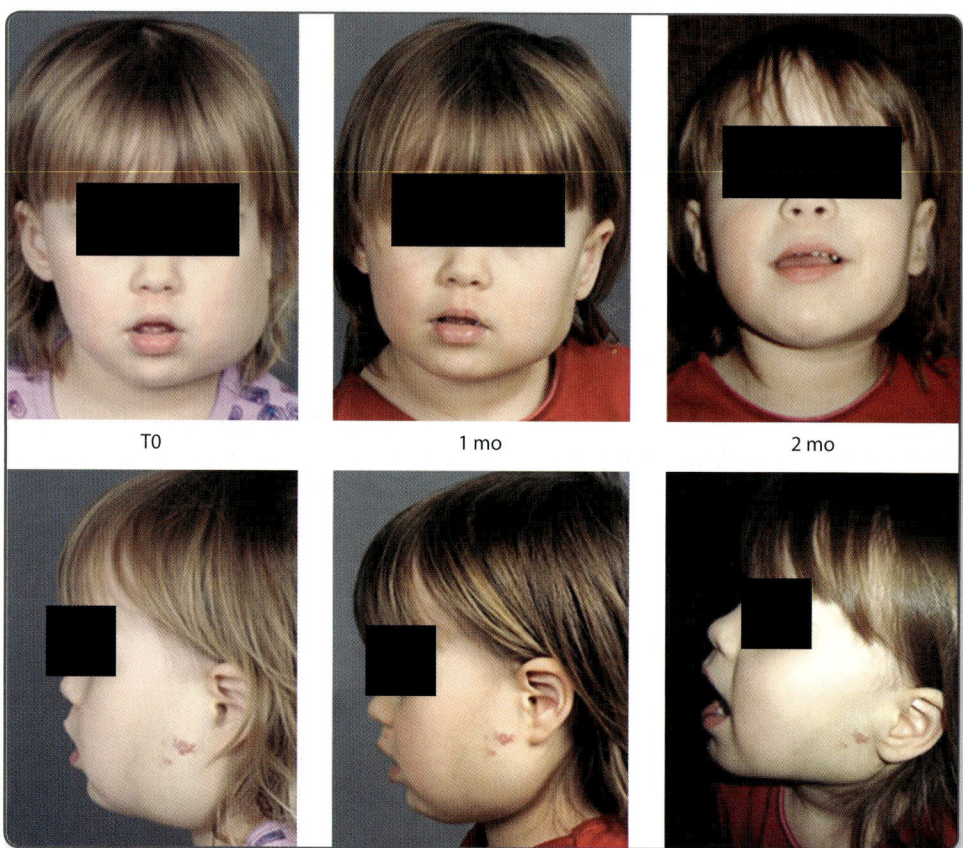

Figure 10.3 Effectiveness of propranolol at involution phase. Propranolol treatment was initiated at the age of 2.5 years in this case of parotid IH.

Side effects

Side effects are uncommon in healthy children.

- Hypoglycaemia is the most dangerous complication. Symptomatic cases, seizures and even one case of death have been reported but overall its prevalence is hard to determine. Cases were often associated with a concomitant infection or poor oral intake, and seem not to be dose related [16,19]
- Bradycardia is usually asymptomatic [4]
- Hypotension
- Bronchial hyper-reactivity
- Nightmares and insomnia are the most frequently encountered side effects
- Acrocyanosis
- Gastrointestinal (GI) disturbances

Parent information

In order to prevent hypoglycaemia, parents have to ensure regular feeding, avoid prolonged fasting and withhold drug administration in case of an acute illness. The only early sign of hypoglycaemia that is not masked by beta-blockade is sweating. Other early signs are shakiness, tachycardia, anxiety and hunger. They should also be taught how to recognise the signs of hypotension and bradycardia.

Special consideration – patients with PHACE syndrome

PHACE is an acronym that stands for posterior fossa brain malformations, segmental haemangiomas of the face or scalp and arterial abnormalities of the head and neck, cardiac anomalies or coarctation of the aorta and eye abnormalities. Theoretically, propranolol may increase the risk of stroke in children with PHACE by inducing hypotension that causes a reduction in already altered cerebral vessels, and by increasing systolic blood pressure variability.

A consensus conference recommends that infants with large facial IH at risk of PHACE undergo a magnetic resonance imaging/angiography of the head, neck and chest including the aorta and an echocardiography. The group that has the highest risk of stroke includes infants with severe, long segment narrowing or no visualisation of major cerebral or cervical arteries, without inadequate collateral circulation, especially when there are coexisting cardiac or aortic anomalies. If a multidisciplinary team including neurology and cardiology agrees that the potential benefits of treatment with propranolol outweigh the risk of stroke, a low dose is initiated and very slowly escalated.

Steroids can be considered as an alternative, but according to the two reported cases of stroke in patients with PHACE syndrome and severe arteriopathy that were under propranolol treatment, the patients were also receiving a steroid treatment.

Acebutolol

A β1 blocker that has been successfully tried as an alternative to propranolol in three papers by French teams. In the first paper [20], it was successful in the treatment of four parotid/facial IHs; in the second paper [15], two out of three subglottic IHs had a favourable response and in the third [4] paper, the success rate was five out of five head and neck lesions. The reason for preferring acebutolol to propranolol which was only detailed in the third paper was insomnia, which is less associated with acebutolol. As a cardioselective drug it could be considered more suitable for cases of bronchial reactivity, but a methodical comparison of its efficacy and safety profile to those of propranolol or steroids is first needed to define its place in the treatment of IH.

Nadolol

A nonselective beta-blocker that has a better safety profile and a longer half-life than propranolol, and is not crossing the blood–brain barrier. One assessor-blinded cohort study [21] enrolling 10 children and comparing photographs at each visit against baseline using a 100-mm visual analogue scale (VAS), found a mean shrinkage of 97% after 24 weeks of Nadolol treatmen The side effects were GI symptoms in five patients (50% of cases), cold extremities in two patients, sleep disturbance in one patient and cold-induced wheezing in one patient.

Timolol

Following the success of propranolol, timolol, a topical nonselective beta-blocker was tried with the intention to avoid the side effects related to the systemic treatment. Several case series reported on a good response of small superficial IH in the proliferative phase to timolol without comparing it to another treatment. One retrospective cohort study [22] gathered the information of 73 infants from five institutions and found that after a mean treatment of 3.4 ± 2.7 months, all patients except one improved, with a mean improvement of 45% measured on a VAS. Another team conducted a randomised placebo-controlled trial enrolling 41 children [23] and found a therapeutic onset of action after 12–16 weeks of therapy, with a significant increase in the number of IH lesions decreasing in size by >5% at weeks 20 and 24. Additionally, a significant decrease in proportional growth rate was noted in the treatment group compared with the placebo group.

Dose

Timolol maleate gel is most commonly used at a concentration of 0.5% applied twice a day. A concentration of 0.1% was used in certain series, but seems to be associated with a lesser tumour response [22]. The use of timolol on mucosal or ulcerated lesions should be subject to caution, as the systemic drug absorption and the resulted effects might be more elevated.

Side effects

The local application of timolol has not been associated with hypotension, hypoglycaemia or any systemic adverse reaction. In the placebo-controlled trial mentioned above, there was no significant variation in blood pressure and heart rate between the groups.

Corticosteroids

For 40 years and up to recently, corticosteroids have been used as the treatment of choice for IH within the proliferative phase and, nowadays, they still have a major role in selected cases.

The response rates reported in the literature are as diverse as the adopted protocols and the definitions used to quantify the effect. Roughly, the rule of third can be applied, i.e. one-third of the lesions respond to the steroidal treatment, one-third respond but stay dependent and one third are resistant [1,24]. In 2001, Bennett et al. [25] systematically reviewed 10 case series, each necessarily including problematic, enlarging cutaneous IH but excluding airway lesions, and found cessation of growth or reduction in the size of the IH in 84% of the patients and a 36% rebound rate.

Regarding IH located in the airway, the rate of response to steroidal treatment is considered higher, approaching 90% [24,26]. A possible explanation is that even a small decrease in the volume of an obstructing tumour or the surrounding inflammation has a dramatic clinical impact.

Dose

The target dose in recent articles is 3 mg/kg per day of prednisone, as a single morning dose [27] to decrease the risk of adrenal suppression. Alternative regimens exist, in which the drug is divided in to three times daily dosing [28], or given on an alternate day basis [26]. As no control trial has compared different regimens, the optimal dose is still to be determined. It does, however, seem as if there were a dose–response relationship [25], but the same equally applies for the side effects.

Duration of treatment

Target dose is usually maintained for a month, followed by a progressive tapering until the end of the proliferative phase, at 9–12 months of age. If the steroidal treatment is given concomitantly to the treatment with propranolol in case of airway lesion, it is usually maintained at a high dose for 1 week and then rapidly discontinued.

Side effects and special considerations

Prolonged steroidal treatment is invariably accompanied by recognised side effects. But, in the treatment of IH, the high dose is usually not maintained long enough to occasion in severe complications such as diabetes, osteoporosis, cataract or glaucoma. The adverse reactions that have been reported in about 35% of the children are reversible and include [25,29]:

- Cushingoid facies, which begins to appear after 1 or 2 months of the treatment
- Personality changes and irritability develop in the first week or two
- Transient growth delay, probably resulting from a temporary inhibition of collagen synthesis
- Transient arterial hypertension
- Gastric irritation

Live attenuated virus vaccine should not be administered during the treatment period. 'Stress doses' of glucocorticoid may be necessary in case of disease or surgery during the time of treatment.

OTHER TREATMENTS

Hypothesising that the renin–angiotensin system has a role in the proliferation of IH, an open-labelled observational clinical trial using captopril, an ACE inhibitor, has been conducted by Tan et al. [30]. Moderate or dramatic response occurred in five out of eight cases during an average treatment period of 10.5 months, with one case of transient elevation of creatinine as the sole complication. Conversely, a retrospective study [31] that analysed cases where captopril was added to treat hypertension that developed during a steroid for IH found that captopril did not sustain the corticosteroid-induced involution.

Interferon and vincristine have been used in the treatment of steroid-resistant cases. However, they were found to be associated with a major toxicity, and are rarely used today.

CONGENITAL HAEMANGIOMA

No treatment is needed for rapidly involuting congenital hemangioma (RICH). As for non involuting congenital hemangioma (NICH), the treatment is usually conservative, although surgical removal associated or not with embolization is sometimes required.

Vascular malformations

Lymphatic malformations

Lymphatic malformations (LMs) are divided into macrocystic, microcystic and mixed types. The macrocystic components are usually defined as cystic spaces identifiable with modern imaging modalities, or as cysts measuring more than 2 cm^3 in volume. Surgery has traditionally been the main treatment for LMs, and is still the preferred choice in some centres for the excision of macrocystic LMs and localized microcystic lesions that are not involving the tongue or the mucosa. Surgery can also be helpful in the debulking of extensive microcystic lesions, or, if using the microdebrider or the coblator, for the reduction in lingual lesions. Nevertheless, it is associated with a considerable recurrence rate (15–53%) [32] and significant morbidity in cases of problematically situated lesions. As invasive radiologists gained experience performing sclerotherapy and elaborated the technique of its use, it has acquired a leading role in the first-line treatment of LMs (**Table 10.3**), either alone or in combination with surgery. With a shift to the use of less toxic drugs, as doxycycline, OK432 and bleomycin, the rate and severity of adverse effects has decreased.

As a general rule for either sclerotherapy or surgery, the treatment of macrocystic LMs is much more successful than for microcystic ones [33]. Indeed, response rates to sclerotherapy, with any of the commonly used agents, often exceed 90% for macrocystic lesions, but remain significantly inferior in cases of mixed or microcystic types.

The combined utilisation of two sclerotherapy agents is an additional option. Shiels et al. [34] treated 16 macrocystic LMs with both sodium tetradecyl sulphate (STS) and ethanol yielding a 100% resolution rate, complicated by infectious cellulitis in two cases. They hypothesise that STS, as a detergent, effectively releases transmembrane lipoproteins from the LM cell membrane, leading to increased membrane permeability and allowing greater membrane penetration of ethanol and doxycycline for intracellular protein denaturation and cell death.

The technique of sclerotherapy involves the aspiration of the macrocysts under ultrasound guidance (US), with a small gauge needle, followed by filling the cysts' space with the chosen sclerosant, at a volume that is smaller than that aspirated [35]. Opacifier can be either injected into the cyst or mixed with the sclerosant to demonstrate communications and extensions. For very large lesions, a pigtail catheter can be installed, the drug is then injected and the drain closed for 12 hours. Repeated drainage and drug injection can be performed over 3 consecutive days, which seems to maximise the effect.

Periprocedural antibiotic or steroid coverage are not routinely necessary, but is mentioned in some publications. The procedure is usually performed under general anaesthesia, although local anaesthesia can be possible in older patients. The endotracheal tube may be left in some cases to protect the airway during the initial swelling. In lesions that do not compromise a vital function and do not entail a disturbing cosmetic defect, observation remains an option as the rate of spontaneous regression is estimated to be 10–15% [36].

OK432

OK432 is a biological product made of cultures of *Streptococcus pyogenes*, treated and killed with penicillin G and then lyophilised. It has immune-enhancing properties by stimulation of the activity of natural killer cells, macrophages and lymphocytes and enhancement of cytokine production. Its quality of sclerosing agent is thought to originate in the strong local inflammation it induces that leads to increased endothelial permeability, accelerated lymph drainage [37] and eventually to fibrosis.

The response of macrocystic type of lesions to OK432 treatment is usually complete or near complete, as shown in a multicentre prospective study by Giguère et al. [38] who found a 86% success rate amongst 22 patients. Similarly, a retrospective study [39] reporting the outcome of 55 patients describes a general long-term response rate of 76%, with the best response rate found amongst macrocystic lesions (92% complete or near complete response). In contrast, the use of sclerotherapy with OK432 on microcystic malformations is more problematic as the effect seems to be restricted mainly to the injected cyst. Hence, the published response rate of microcystic lesions in the above-mentioned papers is 0% and 62% respectively, which is in agreement with the rest of the literature. This partial response can still be of use in some circumstances, as in a preoperative setting, since the impression is that OK432 sclerotherapy does not compromise subsequent surgery.

Dose

The dilution used is 0.01 mg/mL of drug in saline, as originally described by Ogita. The maximum injected amount per session is 0.2 mg. The immediate effect consists of an inflammatory response associated with swelling, erythema, pain and low-grade fever occurs in all patients and resolves within 6 days. The therapeutic response takes about 6 weeks or more and intervals of 6–8 weeks are observed in between the injections.

Contraindications

Penicillin allergy: it is important to note that since OK432 is cultivated in bovine serum, it has been banned in several countries, including Canada, for fear of the Creutzfeldt–Jacob disease.

Side effects

Most reports do not mention adverse reactions beyond the expected initial reaction. In one paper [36], 11% of the injected patients suffered from pain and swelling greater than the routinely expected, but none of the 37 patients had a serious side effect. Another paper [38] describes the following three cases of major events in a total of 22 patients – one case of intracystic haemorrhage 4 weeks after the injection that required an orbital decompression, second case of cervical cellulitis 4–5 weeks after the injection that required intravenous (IV) antibiotherapy and third case of stridor and impending airway obstruction in a patient with a massive LM with an intrathoracic extension.

Doxycycline

Doxycycline is an antibiotic from the tetracycline group that is being used for sclerotherapy of LM for 20 years. Its mechanism of action involves deposition of fibrin and collagen, thus creating fibrosis and adhesions. It inhibits matrix metalloproteinases, cell proliferation, and suppresses the growth of blood and lymph vessels that is induced by VEGF [40,41]. The reported success rates [32,42-44] for the treatment of macrocystic disease are above 90%, around 80% for mixed type and lower with microcystic lesions.

Dose

Doxycycline comes as a lyophilised powder in a 100 mg bottle to which 5 mL of contrast medium and 5 mL of NaCl serum (10 mg/mL) are added. The maximum doses are generally 150 mg in neonates, and up to 1000 mg in older children.

Blood doxycycline levels post-treatment were measured by two teams [32,42], and were found to reach up to 20 times the upper limit of normal. Given that adverse reactions associated with the use of tetracycline occurred in some of the patients, one of the teams [32] changed their practice for the treatment of neonatal lesions by limiting the dose of doxycycline at each instillation to a maximum of 150 mg.

Side effects

The reported complication rates range from 0% to 46% and include [32,41-46]:
- Pain that persists after the normal 2–3 hours, swelling, skin ulceration
- Neural damage
  - Cahill et al. [32] reported on seven cases (14%) of neural damage, all attributed to compression by extensive LMs, six of which self-resolved and one required surgery. The authors cite animal studies in which doxycycline adjacent to a nerve (in contrast to intraepineural injection) was not neurotoxic, and recommend its use, rather than ethanol, in proximity to important nerves
  - Horner's syndrome has also been reported, self-resolving and associated with dysphagia in one case [46]
- Hypoglycaemia, metabolic acidosis and haemolytic anaemia are all known side effects of tetracycline

Bleomycin

Bleomycin is a glycopeptide antibiotic produced by the bacterium *Streptomyces verticillus* that is used as an anticancer agent for its ability to induce breaks in the DNA strands. When injected to a vascular malformation, it destroys the endothelial lining and produces local inflammation and fibrosis.

It can be used as a sclerotherapy agent in the treatment of macrocystic LMs, with a 45% success rate for achieving >90% resolution [47]. However, its major advantage is in microcystic lesions, where aspiration of the cysts content is not feasible. In that case, bleomycin can be directly instilled using a small needle, under US or fluoroscopic guidance [35]. Yang et al. [48] reviewed 65 patients treated with bleomycin A5, isolated from *Streptomyces pingyangensisn* cultures, with success rates, for achieving >90% reduction, of 81% of macrocystic and 63% of microcystic LMs.

Dose

The dilution used is 1 International Unit (IU)/mL of bleomycin in saline. At each session, the total injected drug is usually limited to ½ IU/kg in children younger than 1 year, and up to 15 IU in others. The maximum cumulative dose is 100 IU.

Side effects

The side effects of belomycine treatment are hardly ever mentioned in published papers. Skin ulceration was found in 5 out of 75 (6.7%) patients treated with bleomycin for various vascular anomalies, but the number of cases occurring specifically in LM patients was not detailed in this study [49]. We did not find any report of pulmonary fibrosis developing after the sclerotherapy of an LM. This complication has been associated with a high cumulative IV dose.

OTHER TREATMENTS

Sildenafil

Sildenafil produces vasodilatation by inhibiting phosphodiesterase type 5, which is selectively distributed within the arterial wall smooth muscle of the lungs and penis. In January 2012, Swetman et al. [50] reported that the size of an LM in a child treated with sildenafil for pulmonary hypertension gradually decreased during the 4 months of treatment. Based on that observation, a pilot study was undertaken by that team and two children with LM were treated with sildenafil for 12 weeks. A significant regression of the LM in both cases was followed by a mild enlargement of the lesion when the drug was discontinued. No adverse effect to the drug was noticed. Despite the promising results, there has only been one additional paper [51] describing a good response to sildenafil in two cases of orbital LM.

Sirolimus (rapamycin)

Sirolimus is a macrolide with antifungal and immunosuppressive properties, introduced 14 years ago, and now commonly used to prevent rejection in organ transplantation and as a coronary stent coating. It directly inhibits a cytosolic receptor, thereby preventing downstream protein synthesis and subsequent cell proliferation and angiogenesis (including lymphangiogenesis), as well as activation of T and B cells by interleukin-2.

Following a case report [52] on a dramatic response to sirolimus in the treatment of a refractory kaposiform haemangioendotheliomas with Kasabach–Merritt phenomenon, Hammill et al. [53] published a retrospective case series of six patients with complicated, life-threatening vascular anomalies who were treated with sirolimus for compassionate use after failing multiple other therapies. All the patients, including four cases of extensive microcystic LMs with effusions, had a good response to therapy and tolerated it well.

This encouraging data is not sufficient to allow wide off-label use of the drug, since many questions regarding the anomalies that will best respond, the durability of the effect and the correct length of treatment are still to be answered [54]. Furthermore, it is an immunosuppressive agent with potentially grave long-term effects in infants and young children. Ongoing clinical trials by the same teams will hopefully address these issues.

VENOUS MALFORMATIONS

Sclerotherapy is the initial treatment of choice for venous malformations (VMs). Other therapeutic options include surgical resection, laser photocoagulation, photodynamic therapy and combinations of these methods. Small, nondisturbing lesions can be treated conservatively, but most will eventually become painful, thus requiring intervention. Other indications for the treatment include aesthetic considerations and GI bleed resulting from the malformation-related coagulopathy.

Existing therapies do not claim to cure VMs. Still, pain control is achieved in the majority of patients, and the shrinkage of lesions is also the general rule, albeit usually only with repeated procedures. The outcome is usually more favourable when the treatment is initiated early in life, when the lesions are smaller. Sclerotherapy is typically performed under general anaesthesia, with constant fluoroscopic and/or US control, to avoid extravasation. The technique's details and complications can be found in a review by Alomari et al. [35].

Sodium tetradecyl sulphate

STS is an anionic surfactant commonly used for sclerotherapy. As a detergent, it releases transmembrane lipoproteins from cell membranes and, as shown by animal experiments, it causes a denudation of endothelium, an inflammatory response, and an organised thrombus leading to permanent luminal occlusion and sclerosis [55].

A 3% concentration is used in liquid form or foam, obtained by exchanging STS and air between two syringes. It is considered to be reliable, effective and relatively safe when compared to ethanol, with regard to systemic complications and neuropathy [56].

Reported side effects of STS sclerotherapy include the tendency to cause hyperpigmentation in up to 30% of the patients, epidermal necrosis upon extravasation of higher concentrations and occasional cases of anaphylaxis [57].

Bleomycin

It is considered to produce less swelling than the other sclerosants, and therefore can be used in sensitive areas. It can be used either as a single agent or as an adjuvant to another sclerosant.

Alcohol

Alcohol, or absolute ethanol, is the most destructive sclerosant and is assumed to have the lowest recurrence rate. It induces significant toxicity to blood cells and the intima by dehydration and protein denaturation, resulting in spasm, thrombosis and ultimately vascular obliteration [55]. It also produces tissue swelling and oedema.

The injection of ethanol is painful and, in most cases, necessitates general anaesthesia. The recommended dose in children is 0.5 mL/kg, up to a maximum of 1 mL/kg per session. Reported side effects of alcohol sclerotherapy include cutaneous necrosis, skin blistering, nerve palsy, respiratory depression, cardiac arrhythmias, seizures, rhabdomyolysis, hypoglycaemia and haemolysis. Cardiac arrest has also been reported.

CONCLUSION

The group of vascular anomalies is very heterogeneous in the pathogenesis, the natural course and the response to treatment. Therefore, the interdisciplinary approach is most suitable for establishing the correct diagnosis and choosing the best treatment.

Propranolol has revolutionised the treatment of IH, the most common type of vascular neoplasm, taking over the place of steroid or surgical therapy in most cases. Clinical trials are still needed to define the correct doses, treatment length and possibly expand the traditional indications.

Systemic treatment of vascular malformations is only at a research stage. Sclerotherapy, however, is increasingly assuming a leading role in the treatment of lymphatic and VMs, as interventional radiologists gain experience in the use of less toxic agents. Surgery, which was not addressed in this chapter, remains the main tool for specific cases.

Key points for clinical practice

- IH is considered a vascular neoplasm as it has a proliferative endothelium and a typical clinical evolution.
- In the head and neck, as opposed to the rest of the body, many IHs are periorificial, obstructing or disfiguring and have to be treated.
- IH rapidly responds to propranolol, with a softening of the mass and a decrease in its blushing, or as a decrease in wheezing and dyspnoea for airway lesion.
- Hypoglycaemia is a rare but potentially dangerous complication of propranolol treatment. Families should be instructed to avoid prolonged fasting and withhold drug administration in case of acute illness.
- LM and other vascular malformations have an inactive endothelium post birth. They slowly grow with the child, unless stimulated by infection or trauma, and never regress.
- Sclerotherapy is the first-line treatment of LMs, either alone or in combination with surgery.
- Macrocystic LMs respond well to most sclerosing agents. Similarly, the surgical treatment of macrocystic LMs yields better results than surgery for microcystic lesions.

REFERENCES

1. Enjolras O, Wassef M, Chapot R. In : Enjolras O (ed), Color Atlas of Vascular Tumors and Vascular Malformations. Cambridge: Cambridge University Press; 2007.
2. Parikh, Darrow DH, Grimmer JF, et al. Propranolol use for infantile hemangiomas. JAMA Otolaryngol Head Neck Surg 2013; 139:153–156.
3. Denoyelle F, Garabédian E.-N. Propranolol may become first-line treatment in obstructive subglottic infantile hemangiomas. Otolaryngol Head Neck Surg 2010; 142:463–464.
4. Fuchsmann C, et al. Propranolol as first-line treatment of head and neck hemangiomas. Arch Otolaryngol Head Neck Surg 2011; 137:471–478.
5. Saint-Jean M, et al. Propranolol for treatment of ulcerated infantile hemangiomas. J Am Acad Dermatol 2011; 64:827–832.
6. Caussé S, et al. Propranolol-resistant infantile haemangiomas. Br J Dermatol 2013; 169:125–129.
7. Hogeling M, Adams S, Wargon O. A randomized controlled trial of propranolol for infantile hemangiomas. Pediatrics 2011; 128:e259–266.
8. Bertrand J, McCuaig C, Dubois J, et al. Propranolol versus prednisone in the treatment of infantile hemangiomas: a retrospective comparative study. Pediatr Dermatol 2011; 28:649–654.

9. Price CJ, et al. Propranolol vs corticosteroids for infantile hemangiomas: a multicenter retrospective analysis. Arch Dermatol 2011; 147:1371–1376.

10. Peridis S, Pilgrim G, Athanasopoulos I, Parpounas K. A meta-analysis on the effectiveness of propranolol for the treatment of infantile airway haemangiomas. Int J Pediatr Otorhinolaryngol 2011; 75:455–460.

11. Lou Y, et al. The effectiveness of propranolol in treating infantile hemangiomas: a meta-analysis including 35 studies. Br J Clin Pharmacol 2013; 78(1):44–57.

12. Hermans DJJ, et al. Propranolol, a very promising treatment for ulceration in infantile hemangiomas: a study of 20 cases with matched historical controls. J Am Acad Dermatol 2011; 64:833–838.

13. Storch CH, Hoeger PH. Propranolol for infantile haemangiomas: insights into the molecular mechanisms of action. Br J Dermatol 2010; 163:269–274.

14. Itinteang T, Brasch HD, Tan ST, Day DJ. Expression of components of the renin-angiotensin system in proliferating infantile haemangioma may account for the propranolol-induced accelerated involution. J Plast Reconstr Aesthet Surg 2011; 64:759–765.

15. Blanchet C, Nicollas R, Bigorre M, Amedro P, Mondain M. Management of infantile subglottic hemangioma: acebutolol or propranolol? Int J Pediatr Otorhinolaryngol 2010; 74:959–961.

16. Drolet BA, et al. Initiation and use of propranolol for infantile hemangioma: report of a consensus conference. Pediatrics 2013; 131:128–140.

17. Bingham MM, Saltzman B, Vo N-J, Perkins JA. Propranolol reduces infantile hemangioma volume and vessel density. Otolaryngol Head Neck Surg 2012; 147:338–344.

18. Janmohamed SR, et al. Scoring the proliferative activity of haemangioma of infancy: the Haemangioma Activity Score (HAS). Clin Exp Dermatol 2011; 36:715–723.

19. Holland KE, et al. Hypoglycemia in children taking propranolol for the treatment of infantile hemangioma. Arch Dermatol 2010; 146:775–778.

20. Bigorre M, Van Kien AK, Valette H. Beta-blocking agent for treatment of infantile hemangioma. Plast Reconstr Surg 2009; 123:195e–196e.

21. Pope E, Chakkittakandiyil A, Lara-Corrales I, Maki E, Weinstein M. Expanding the therapeutic repertoire of infantile haemangiomas: cohort-blinded study of oral nadolol compared with propranolol. Br J Dermatol 2013; 168:222–224.

22. Chakkittakandiyil A, et al. Timolol maleate 0.5% or 0.1% gel-forming solution for infantile hemangiomas: a retrospective, multicenter, cohort study. Pediatr Dermatol 2012; 29:28–31.

23. Chan H, McKay C, Adams S, Wargon O. RCT of timolol maleate gel for superficial infantile hemangiomas in 5- to 24-week-olds. Pediatrics 2013; 131:e1739–1747.

24. Herbreteau D, Robier A, Disant F. In: Romanet P (ed), Pathologie Vasculaire en ORL. Paris: Société Francaise d'ORL et de Chirurgie de la Face et du Cou, 2000.

25. Bennett ML, Fleischer AB, Chamlin SL, Frieden IJ. Oral corticosteroid use is effective for cutaneous hemangiomas: an evidence-based evaluation. Arch Dermatol 2001; 137:1208–1213.

26. Hawkins DB, Crockett DM, Kahlstrom EJ, MacLaughlin EF. Corticosteroid management of airway hemangiomas: long-term follow-up. Laryngoscope 1984; 94:633–637.

27. Greene AK, Couto RA. Oral prednisolone for infantile hemangioma: efficacy and safety using a standardized treatment protocol. Plast Reconstr Surg. 2011; 128:743–752.

28. Nieuwenhuis K, de Laat PCJ, Janmohamed SR, Madern GC, Oranje AP. Infantile hemangioma: treatment with short course systemic corticosteroid therapy as an alternative for propranolol. Pediatr Dermatol 2013; 30:64–70.

29. Greene AK. Systemic corticosteroid is effective and safe treatment for problematic infantile hemangioma. Pediatr Dermatol 2010; 27:322–323.

30. Tan ST, et al. Treatment of infantile haemangioma with captopril. Br J Dermatol 2012; 167:619–624.

31. Christou EM, Wargon O. Effect of captopril on infantile haemangiomas: a retrospective case series. Australas J Dermatol 2012; 53:216–218.

32. Cahill AM, et al. Percutaneous sclerotherapy in neonatal and infant head and neck lymphatic malformations: a single center experience. J Pediatr Surg 2011; 46:2083–2095.

33. Perkins, JA, Chen, EY. In: Flint PW et al editors. Cummings Otolaryngology: Head and Neck Surgery. 5th ed. Philadelphia: Elsevier; 2010.

34. Shiels WE, Kenney BD, Caniano DA, Besner GE. Definitive percutaneous treatment of lymphatic malformations of the trunk and extremities. J Pediatr Surg 2008; 43:136–9; discussion 140.

35. Alomari A, Dubois J. Interventional management of vascular malformations. Tech Vasc Interv Radiol 2011; 14:22–31.

36. Boardman SJ, Cochrane LA, Roebuck D, Elliott MJ, Hartley BEJ. Multimodality treatment of pediatric lymphatic malformations of the head and neck using surgery and sclerotherapy. Arch Otolaryngol Head Neck Surg 2010; 136:270–276.
37. Ogita S, et al. OK-432 therapy for lymphangioma in children: why and how does it work? J Pediatr Surg 1996; 31:477–480.
38. Giguère CM, et al. Treatment of lymphangiomas with OK-432 (Picibanil) sclerotherapy: a prospective multi-institutional trial. Arch Otolaryngol Head Neck Surg 20002; 128:1137–1144.
39. Yoo JC, et al. OK-432 sclerotherapy in head and neck lymphangiomas: long-term follow-up result. Otolaryngol Head Neck Surg 2009; 140:120–123.
40. Hurewitz AN, Lidonicci K, Wu CL, Reim D, Zucker S. Histologic changes of doxycycline pleurodesis in rabbits. Effect of concentration and pH. Chest. 1994; 106:1241–1245.
41. Shergill A, John P, Amaral JG. Doxycycline sclerotherapy in children with lymphatic malformations: outcomes, complications and clinical efficacy. Pediatr Radiol 2012; 42:1080–1088.
42. Burrows PE, et al. Percutaneous sclerotherapy of lymphatic malformations with doxycycline. Lymphat Res Biol 2008; 6:209–216.
43. Alomari AI, Karian VE, Lord DJ, Padua HM, Burrows PE. Percutaneous sclerotherapy for lymphatic malformations: a retrospective analysis of patient-evaluated improvement. J Vasc Interv Radiol 2006; 17:1639–1648.
44. Nehra D, et al. Doxycycline sclerotherapy as primary treatment of head and neck lymphatic malformations in children. J Pediatr Surg 2008; 43:451–460.
45. Molitch HI, Unger EC, Witte CL, VanSonnenberg E. Percutaneous sclerotherapy of lymphangiomas. Radiology 1995; 194:343–347.
46. Wang KL, Chun RH, Kerschner JE, Sulman CG. Sympathetic neuropathy and dysphagia following doxycycline sclerotherapy. Int J Pediatr Otorhinolaryngol 2013; 77:1613–1616.
47. Churchill P, et al. Sclerotherapy for lymphatic malformations in children: a scoping review. J Pediatr Surg 2011; 46:912–922.
48. Yang Y, et al. Bleomycin A5 sclerotherapy for cervicofacial lymphatic malformations. J Vasc Surg 2011; 53:150–155.
49. Hassan Y, Osman AK, Altyeb A. Noninvasive management of hemangioma and vascular malformation using intralesional bleomycin injection. Ann Plast Surg 2013; 70:70–73.
50. Swetman GL, et al. Sildenafil for severe lymphatic malformations. N Engl J Med 2012; 366:384–386.
51. Gandhi NG, Lin LK, O'Hara M. Sildenafil for pediatric orbital lymphangioma. JAMA Ophthalmol. 2013; 131:1228–1230.
52. Blatt J, Stavas J, Moats-Staats B, Woosley J, Morrell DS. Treatment of childhood kaposiform hemangioendothelioma with sirolimus. Pediatr Blood Cancer 2010; 55:1396–1398.
53. Hammill AM, Wentzel MS, Nelson S, et al. Sirolimus for the treatment of complicated vascular anomalies in children. 2011;57(6):1018–1024.
54. Trenor CC. Sirolimus for refractory vascular anomalies. Pediatr Blood Cancer 2011; 57:904–905.
55. Albanese G, Kondo KL. Pharmacology of sclerotherapy. Semin Intervent Radiol 2010; 27:391–399.
56. Burrows PE. Endovascular treatment of slow-flow vascular malformations. Tech Vasc Interv Radiol 2013; 16:12–21.
57. Brzoza Z, Kasperska-Zajac A, Rogala E, Rogala B. Anaphylactoid reaction after the use of sodium tetradecyl sulfate: a case report. Angiology 2007; 58(5):644–646.

Index

Note: Page numbers in **bold** or *italic* refer to tables or figures, respectively.